VICTORY OVER MIGRAINE

The Breakthrough Study That Explains What Causes It and How It Can Be Completely Prevented

by
Professor Rodolfo Low

with an introduction by
Fredric W. Pullen II, M.D.

An Owl Book   Henry Holt and Company   New York

Henry Holt and Company, Inc.
Publishers since 1866
115 West 18th Street
New York, New York 10011

Henry Holt® is a registered trademark
of Henry Holt and Company, Inc.

Published in Canada by Fitzhenry & Whiteside Ltd.,
195 Allstate Parkway, Markham, Ontario L3R 4T8.

Library of Congress Cataloging-in-Publication Data
Low, Rodolfo.
[Migraine]
Victory over migraine: the breakthrough study that explains what
causes it and how it can be completely prevented / by Rodolfo Low;
with an introduction by Fredric W. Pullen II.—1st Owl Book ed.
        p.   cm.
Originally published under the title: Migraine, 1987.
"An Owl book."
Includes index.
Bibliography: p.
1. Migraine—Diet therapy—Popular works.
2. Migraine—Prevention—Popular works.   3. Sugar-free diet.
I. Title.
RC392.L69   1989   88-38990
616.8'57—dc19   CIP

ISBN 0-8050-0927-2 (An Owl Book: pbk.)

Henry Holt books are available for special promotions and premiums.
For details contact: Director, Special Markets.

First published in hardcover as *Migraine* by
Henry Holt and Company, Inc., in 1987.

First Owl Book Edition—1989

Designed by Kate Nichols
Printed in the United States of America

10   9   8   7   6

To my wife

*The research
upon which this book is based
was partially financed by two grants
from the Ford Foundation.*

Contents

Foreword

In late 1982 I met Professor Rodolfo Low, and by coincidence our conversation led us to a subject of common interest. For many years I have been interested in the relationship of blood sugar levels to Ménière's disease—an ailment characterized by recurring episodes of severe dizziness, hearing loss, and noises in the ear. Professor Low devoted twenty years of his life to proving that migraine headaches are directly related to blood sugar levels and that in genetically predisposed people they are a consequence of an overactive pancreas. The excess insulin produced by this endocrine gland enhances the secretion of opposing hormones, the catecholamines, which in turn stimulate the production of vasodilating prostaglandins that initiate the migraine attack.

I must confess that I was very skeptical about his theory. He showed me a series of charts indicating high insulin production in dozens of migraine sufferers whom he had advised for relief of the headaches. He emphatically stated that migraine headaches can be prevented by a diet rich in natural carbohydrates—I repeat rich, not poor, as is so frequently recommended in diets to control hypoglycemia. The diet, however, must be completely devoid of refined sugar, and meals must be taken at prescribed intervals according to a strict timetable. The regimen is not difficult. Professor Low stated that over 90 percent of the true migraine sufferers who strictly followed his advice have been relieved of their misery permanently.

This was hard to believe, so I proposed that he come to the United States and repeat his research in our laboratory under the auspices of the Hearing Education and Research Foundation. The foundation is involved in basic research of the cause of dizziness and hearing loss. It has been well known for many years that migraine headache and Ménière's disease are associated in many patients; and this relationship needed to be further investigated. We have now studied this problem for three years, and I must state we have now replicated his research in our own patients, including many who had not found relief through the standard medical migraine treatment they had received during years of suffering.

This book relates the history of Professor Low's experience and research, and gives a clear accounting of his findings, illuminated with interesting case histories. It is presented for critical analysis and to stimulate further research, and also to serve as a practical guide to help sufferers eliminate their migraine headaches.

Professor Low's results are indeed astonishing, and his experimentally proven theory is logical and easy to understand. What is less easy to understand is why none of the many organizations all over the world devoted exclusively to research on migraine did not reach the same conclusion earlier. It seems to be a common belief in the sciences that difficult questions always have difficult answers, and so the most simple channels of exploration are often ignored. Professor Low has found what turns out to be a relatively simple answer to a difficult question. And most important, he makes clear that it is also relatively simple for individuals suffering from migraine to eliminate it from their lives.

Fredric W. Pullen II, M.D.
President
Hearing Education and
Research Foundation
Miami, Florida

Introduction

The twentieth century has indeed been a golden era in medicine. The discovery of penicillin in 1928 by Alexander Fleming has, by itself, added years to the human life span. Before the introduction of antibiotics, a pus-filled cut or scratch was serious enough to warrant alarm, and the pneumococcus bacteria annually felled thousands of its unfortunate victims. Tuberculosis, the dreaded killer of past generations, can now be arrested by treatment with new "wonder" drugs such as streptomycin, isoniazid, and para-aminosalicylic acid. X rays and skin testing are valuable for early detection. Insulin therapy has provided the once doomed diabetic the opportunity to live a relatively normal life. Mothers of the 1940s and 1950s were ever watchful for signs of the widespread crippler poliomyelitis. Who among us old enough to remember can ever forget the relentless warnings of the "polio season"? "Be careful, don't catch a chill." "Don't overtire yourself." "Avoid that swim in the neighborhood pool." Fortunately, these warnings are only memories now. Since the advent of the Salk and Sabin vaccines and their continued use, poliomyelitis has been practically wiped out. Organ transplants are routinely executed, and now life can even be generated in an artificial environment outside of the mother's womb.

In 1900 the life expectancy in the United States was 47.9 years for males and 51.1 years for females. The estimate for 1984 was 71.1 years for males and 78.3 years for females, an increase of approximately 48 percent for males and 52 percent for females. All indicators point to a continued rise in life expectancies, with an even greater increase forecast as advances are made in treating cardiovascular disease and cancer.

Consequently, there should be a very bright future in store for this generation and those that follow.

Nevertheless, many unanswered questions still plague the medical establishment, questions to which they can only respond, "We don't know" or "Let's try this." Even more frustrating for the patient is the overused reply, "It's probably just your nerves." How many of us have been told to take a vacation or change jobs as a solution for inexplicable aches and pains? We probably won't die from these discomforts, but they will do much over the years to diminish our well-being and peace of mind.

It is to those who suffer from just such a disorder that this book is addressed. Migraine is not "a mysterious headache" for which there is no hope. This book outlines an easy procedure that will bring complete and permanent relief to persons afflicted with this problem—a problem commonly considered beyond our present knowledge. Although it presents the pertinent scientific facts, the text is written in simple language so that the layman can comprehend its message without difficulty.

Many new concepts are presented in these pages, especially the body mechanism that is responsible for a migraine attack. Much of what is discussed here has actually been known for many years, though remarkably it has been overlooked by other researchers. The story begins in 1922 with the discovery of insulin—a hormone produced by the pancreas that alleviates the symptoms of diabetes. Diabetics have a higher-than-normal blood sugar level, a condition known as *hyperglycemia*, which is a direct result of the failure of the pancreas to produce sufficient insulin. Injecting the patient with insulin restores his blood sugar level to normal. The disease is not cured, but its symptoms subside.

The use of insulin, however, involves certain dangers. An excessive dose of this hormone causes the blood sugar to fall below normal, a condition called *hypoglycemia*. This condition generates a series of exceedingly unpleasant symptoms that in extreme cases, if sufficient glucose is not administered promptly, can result in the patient's death.

Only two years after the discovery of insulin, Seale Harris, a professor at the University of Alabama, noted that a number of individuals spontaneously presented symptoms similar to those of diabetics who had received an overdose of insulin. In these cases, however, the characteristic symptoms were caused by an overactive pancreas, which produced too much insulin and caused the blood sugar to drop below normal. Harris termed this condition hyperinsulinism, and published his observations in 1924 in the *Journal of the American Medical Association*.

As described in this book, it is of fundamental importance that particular products, especially but not only refined sugar, can stimulate the production of an abnormally high level of insulin in individuals whose pancreas is overactive, causing hypoglycemia.

It should be mentioned that in modern medical language the use of the word *hypoglycemia* is limited to specific conditions, especially to those in which the lowest blood sugar levels are simultaneous with the strongest symptoms. When these conditions are not met, as in the case of migraine headache, the term *idiopathic postprandial syndrome* is used instead. As it is only a matter of semantics, the word *hypoglycemia* will be used throughout this book, as well as the word *hyperinsulinism* which is the most frequent cause of low blood sugar.

In literature on hypoglycemia, headache is repeatedly cited as a symptom. The specific term *migraine*, however, was not associated in early publications with blood sugar levels, but later several papers were published showing that such a relationship actually exists. In one paper published in 1949 in the *American Journal of the Medical Sciences*, Professor C. F. Wilkinson, Jr., of the University of Michigan, even suggested that the term *migraine* be abandoned and that *hypoglycemic headache* be used instead.

Here then was the key to preventing migraine attacks. Unfortunately, for many reasons, this exciting hypothesis was forgotten. There was much disagreement over the specific treatment for hyperinsulinism. Some authors recommended a diet rich in protein and without carbohydrates, while others insisted on one that was high in carbohydrates. Research proceeded in other directions and the opportunity to pursue this avenue of research and bring relief to individuals suffering from migraine was lost. The purpose of this book is to remedy that error.

The many years I have devoted to research in this field grew out of a personal need: I simply decided not to suffer with this incapacitating disease any longer, to find an explanation and cure for it. Happily, I succeeded, and it is my desire to help the millions of other migraine sufferers free themselves as well. I would also like to make doctors who treat migraine aware of the results of my experiments and of the clinical application that will eliminate the distress of migraine.

The case histories presented in the book are genuine, but the names are fictitious. There is one exception to this and that is the name of Dr. George Villabona, my friend and medical doctor who motivated me to initiate my research on migraine headache.

I would not like to conclude this introduction without expressing my gratitude to Fredric W. Pullen II, M.D., who invited me to come to the United States to repeat the research I had done elsewhere, and to both B. Todd Troost, M.D., Chairman of the Department of Neurology, and Larry A. Pearce, M.D., Associate Professor of Neurology, Bowman Gray School of Medicine, Wake Forest University, Winston-Salem, North Carolina, for testing and proving the validity of my procedure to relieve migraine headache.

I am also especially indebted to Nelson Buhler for his assistance in getting this book published; to Maria C. Casas, who performed thousands of laboratory tests for me in connection with this work; to Norton Canfield, M.D., who worked closely with me and gave me all necessary assistance to bring this endeavor to a successful conclusion; and to Carol A. Albright for her invaluable help in the development of the manuscript.

Professor Rodolfo Low

Victory over Migraine

1

A Case History

On a cool July evening in 1968, my wife and I were the guests of Professor Edward Lynch and his wife, Dorothy, at the first public concert given by their daughter, Anna. We had met the professor several months before, and Anna's great skill as a pianist was well known to us. Professor Lynch was in high spirits, beaming with fatherly pride as he greeted familiar faces. Many friends and members of the family were in attendance for Anna's debut, and so the concert hall was nearly full when we arrived.

Dorothy Lynch looked tense—probably worried, I thought, that her daughter would not be well accepted.

"She is so nervous," said Dorothy, "and one of her headaches was beginning when she left the house tonight. She's just like me. I always suffer from migraine when I get upset. Sometimes it lasts for two days."

"Oh?" I said, showing my professional interest. "I've done quite a bit of research on the cause of migraine headache,

you know. Perhaps we could talk about this sometime."
Dorothy nodded politely but with obvious disinterest, and
fixed her eyes on the enormity of the yet-empty stage.

Red velvet framed a shimmering gold backdrop, but the
stately grand piano was the center of attention. In just a
few minutes, Anna would sit there, alone and small, and,
as we all anticipated, would give a magnificent performance.

The lights dimmed and a hush traveled to the back of the
theater as Anna walked onto the stage. Applause filled the
concert hall, Professor Lynch's hands contributing loudly.
Anna seated herself with the dignity expected of a serious
artist. She looked lovely, though very young for one so
talented.

She began the first number on the program, and her
hands danced over the keyboard, filling the hall with a familiar and beautiful piece. She performed Beethoven's So-
nata in F minor, op. 57, no. 23 ("Appassionata"), expertly,
and as she played, I closed my eyes and lost myself in the
music. Anna was doing very well indeed, and I thought,
Dorothy, you have no need to worry about your daughter
tonight. This is her shining moment.

When she had only a few minutes remaining, however,
before completing the selection, the sound quite suddenly
changed. The pace slowed. Was she drifting into her second
number? I glanced down at my program. No. It soon became
obvious that Anna was making quite a few mistakes.

We listened for more than a minute to the hesitations of
a beginner trying to get the number right. Anna looked
confused and now appeared to be playing with only one
hand. Her right hand was perched immobile on the keyboard, as if frozen in that position. The audience looked on
incredulously and, after a while, began to stir.

Anna stopped, rose slowly, and stumbled from the stage.

"Oh, what a shame," my wife whispered to me. "She must be so embarrassed "

After a moment of disbelief, the professor and Dorothy stood. Polite smiles did not mask their disappointment and shock.

"I'm sorry, I don't understand," Professor Lynch apologized. "We really must go to Anna now " My wife and I hurried close behind them, away from a questioning crowd.

When we arrived backstage, Anna sat on the steps that had led from her musical disaster. She held her head with both hands.

"The pain is so bad!" she said. "I couldn't see the keyboard. The spots were there again I could only see the spots." Anna was on the verge of hysteria, crying and holding on to her mother.

Later, when Anna was at home and had calmed down somewhat, she explained further: "I just couldn't remember the end of the piece! Can you believe it?" She looked sadly at her father.

"But Anna," the professor noted, "you knew it perfectly. You've practiced it for years."

Anna began to whimper again as she held an ice bag to her throbbing head, but continued, "Finally, I had no feeling in my hand. This one " She held up her right hand. "After that I just panicked. I couldn't remember anything."

We all sat in silence for a few minutes, trying to digest what had happened. I then inquired, "Anna, would you mind if I ask you some questions?"

"No, of course not, Professor Low."

"How long have you suffered from migraines?"

"Since I was fourteen, I think. About five years." Her mother nodded in agreement. "Sometimes I get nauseous with them. I used to miss so much school"

"Have you experienced this loss of feeling before?"

"Yes, but it isn't always my hand. My face gets numb and I usually lose some of the feeling in my tongue."

"And the figures you see? Are these part of your attacks?"

"Oh, yes, almost always. I thought I was going to get a spell tonight. I could feel it coming on, and then I saw the spots! It was horrible."

These were all common symptoms of migraine headache. We left Anna to rest for a few minutes and I talked to her parents to see what treatment, if any, their daughter had received. They explained that she had been seen by a number of specialists, all of whom eventually attributed her condition to tension. Anna was told that she would simply have to get her nerves under control, and was given a variety of tranquilizers over the years to take on a regular basis. She even had a prescription with her that night. But these medicines did not seem to decrease the intensity or the frequency of her migraine attacks. At the suggestion of the family physician, Anna had seen a well-known psychoanalyst, who felt that the source of her migraine could be directly traced to subconscious conflicts originating in an inferiority complex. According to this specialist, who probably belonged to the Adler school,* this feeling of inferiority motivated her to excel as a pianist. Visits to his office had lasted for over two years, but Anna did not experience any improvement.

"No, no." I shook my head. "This is neither a mental nor an emotional disease. It is definitely a biochemical disorder and should be treated as such. Anna, what have you had to eat today?"

---

*Alfred Adler (1870–1937) was a psychiatrist who developed a psychotherapy to direct those disabled by inferiority feelings toward social usefulness.

"Oh, nothing at all really. Just a Coke and a piece of cake. I was too nervous to eat very much."

"Um-hmm. And that is precisely what started all of your trouble this evening. Anna, how would you like to be rid of your migraines for good?"

By now everyone was staring at me, but my wife smiled knowingly. I then made what must have seemed a very bold statement: "If Anna will follow my instructions, she will never have another attack of migraine."

Anna has given many successful performances since that night in 1968. She is critically acclaimed as one of the most accomplished pianists in the country. Many demands are made on her daily, both as an artist and as one who has earned the support of thousands of devoted and admiring fans. And yet in eighteen years Anna has not had one attack of migraine. She has acquired greater self-confidence and emotional stability, as well as a sense of physical health that was previously unknown to her. Anna's mother, Dorothy, delighted by the improvement in her daughter, followed her child's example, and both are now completely free of the symptoms of this disorder.

2

What Is a Migraine?

The earliest detailed descriptions of migraine are those written by the Greek physician and philosopher Claudius Galen (131–201) and by Aretaeus the Cappadocian, who lived in the second century. It is curious that neither of these authors mentions the other in his writings, although both refer to eminent medical authorities of an earlier age. It is therefore generally thought that the two were rivals, though the record is not completely clear on this point. Hippocrates, the "father of medicine," who had practiced six hundred years before, was a model for both men, and they brought about a revival of his teachings. It should be noted that Hippocrates, although he wrote elaborately about many other disorders such as tuberculosis, plague, and lobar pneumonia, did not mention migraine anywhere in his works. It is probable that migraine did not exist during or before his time.

Galen was born in Pergamum, a city in Asia Minor, and

wrote his *Treatise on Medical Experience* before he had reached the age of twenty-one. He traveled to Rome and practiced in the court of the emperor, Marcus Aurelius, at which time he penned many of his voluminous medical theories. Galen wrote on such diverse subjects as natural faculties, hygiene, anatomy, sense and perception, and disease. He was quite knowledgeable in his anatomical descriptions and is credited with founding experimental physiology. It was Claudius Galen who first used the term *hemicrania*, from which the word *migraine* derived.

Aretaeus was a native of the hilly country of Asia Minor above the Euphrates River and practiced his trade in Alexandria and Rome. His descriptions of diseases are amazingly detailed and accurate for the era in which he lived. It was Aretaeus who first described tetanus, epilepsy, and the murmur of heart disease. He also gave us the first account of diabetes and is responsible for suggesting its name. He wrote: "The fluid uses the patient's body as a ladder to escape downward." The Greek word for ladder is *diabaition*.

The writings of Aretaeus were lost for many centuries, but in 1552 they fell into the hands of Junius Paulus Crassus, who first translated them from the original Greek into Latin. From the later English translation by Francis Adams, published in 1856, we find Aretaeus's description of migraine, under the heading Cephalaea:

. . . and in certain cases the whole head is pained; and the pain is sometimes on the right and sometimes on the left side, or the forehead, or the bregma; and these may all occur the same day in a random manner.

But in certain cases, the parts on the right side, or on the left solely, so far that a separate temple, or ear, or one eyebrow, or one eye, or the nose which divides the face into two equal parts; and the pain does not pass this limit, but remains in the half of the head. This is called *Heterocrania*, an illness by no means mild, even though it intermits, and although it appears slight. For if at any time it sets in acutely, it occasions unseemly and dreadful symptoms: spasm and distortion of the countenance take place; the eyes either fixed intently like horns, or they are rolled inwardly to this side or that; vertigo; deep-seated pain of the eyes as far as the meninges; irre-strainable sweat; sudden pain of the tendons, as of one striking with a club; nausea; vomiting of bilious matters; collapse of the patient . . . the patients, moreover, are weary of life, and wish to die.

Migraine headache, then, has been known for close to two thousand years, and throughout history we find men-tion of the disease in both technical and fictional literature. In a treatise by Felix Wuertz, a Swiss physician born be-tween 1500 and 1510, he admits that he once suffered an attack of hemicrania that lasted for ten days, and experi-enced relief only after an arteriotomy was performed upon his left temporal artery. This was not an uncommon practice in severe migraine, it seems, since the pain can be unbear-able and the patient is willing to try anything for its abate-ment. This was at best, however, an excessive measure that could provide only temporary relief.

How many Victorian heroines were confined to their beds with either real or imaginary attacks of migraine? You will recall that feigning a migraine is always a convenient way for a fictional character to avoid an unpleasant confronta-tion. It is no coincidence that the other characters unques-tioningly accept the victim's complete incapacity when he chooses this as an excuse. Migraine has no easy cure.

Just what is a migraine? The name *migraine* is given to a recurrent, throbbing headache of variable duration, intensity, and frequency, a headache that is often preceded by visual disturbances and accompanied by irritability, aversion to light and sound, nausea, and occasionally vomiting. Textbooks of medicine usually separate migraines into different types. These classifications have, however, no practical application, since all forms of the disease have one common cause.

Often the victims of migraine are aware of the approach of an attack before the initiation of the headache. They might experience a feeling of languor or sleepiness. Later they have the impression of seeing only half of all objects, a phenomenon known as *hemianopsia*. They will probably see spots of different shapes and colors moving before their eyes. These scintillating spots, called *scotomas*, vary in size and shape from specks to clearly delineated geometric figures. Sometimes they are dull, while other times they may possess an extraordinary brilliance. Although normally black and white, they have appeared in every imaginable color.

When the actual pain begins, it is usually localized in the temple or in the eyeball on one side of the head. Occasionally it spreads downward to the neck and, in rare instances, to the arm. The sensation is one of intense, throbbing pain that is aggravated by exposure to light, noise, or movement. Many patients become worse when standing or sitting, but in some cases the condition intensifies when they lie down. There is usually some nausea, but actual vomiting seldom occurs. Some individuals also experience intense cold.

In severe cases, patients have tingling sensations and lose sensibility in the lips, the tongue, and sometimes the face or fingers of the hand on the side of the body affected by the headache.

Finally, a migraine victim is frequently beset by mental confusion and difficulty in speaking. Loss of sensibility and mental confusion can occur either before or at the onset of the headache. Speech problems almost always occur only after the actual pain has begun. In such a case, the patient knows what he wants to say but is incapable of expressing it. Often he says something entirely different from what he had intended. Moreover, he is completely aware of the error. In the most extreme cases of migraine, real amnesia can occur at the height of an attack. All symptoms disappear at the end of the seizure, which can vary in length from a few minutes to several days.

Of course, not all persons suffering from migraine experience all of the same symptoms. Visual disturbances can be the only discomfort in some cases. In others, the headache can begin with no warning. Although the pain is usually unilateral (hence Galen's name of *hemicrania* for the disease), there have been cases where it has spread to the entire head. Not only do the precise details of a migraine vary from one person to another, but the same person can have dissimilar attacks on different occasions.

In his work *Migraine: Clinical Features, Mechanisms and Management* (1969), J. Pearce gives interesting statistical data regarding the age at which migraine attacks usually begin in life. These data were assembled by several researchers, and the conclusions reached are the following:

1. In one-third of all cases the onset of the condition occurred before the age of ten.
2. Fifty-six percent of all migraine patients had their first attack by the age of sixteen.
3. In 90 percent of the cases the initial attack occurred before the age of forty.

About 5 percent of all children suffer from some type of regular headaches, which are usually migraines. In early childhood, however, the symptoms of migraine may not always include an actual headache but are migrainous in origin, consisting of intermittent vomiting, a sensitivity to movement, and sometimes feelings of inexplicable weakness and intense hunger. As puberty approaches, migraine attacks become more common among children who have the congenital predisposition for them, and can generally be differentiated from other disorders. It is unusual for the disease to commence after one has reached midlife, but there have been some such cases. It appears, then, that migraine has its onset at a relatively young age. The above observations therefore tend to discredit the popularly held theory that the disease occurs predominantly in persons who are perfectionists or who exhibit a rigidity of behavior. Traits such as these are basically learned and become more deeply ingrained as life goes on. My personal experience is that perfectionists are mainly found among middle-aged and elderly people but only seldom among youngsters. Therefore, if perfectionism were indeed a legitimate cause of the disease, the data would read in reverse: the number of initial attacks would climb with age.

Although migraine has been known for almost two thousand years, it was only in the nineteenth century that serious studies of the disease were undertaken. Several investigators found that most of its symptoms are due to a change in the caliber of the blood vessels in the head. They discovered that a reduction of the diameter of these vessels, called *vasoconstriction*, takes place at the beginning of an attack, simultaneous with the visual disturbances. This is followed by a widening of the caliber of the blood vessels, or *vasodilation*, which coincides with the beginning of the pain.

A number of treatises of that time cite long periods of fasting as one of migraine's causes and mention that for some persons several hours without eating is enough to bring on an attack. This would seem to suggest that hypoglycemia produced migraine, although at the time nothing was yet known about blood sugar levels. After the discovery of insulin in 1922 by Best and Banting, an interest was stirred in a newly described disease, hypoglycemia. Dr. Seale Harris of the University of Alabama noticed that several patients who were not diabetic and therefore not taking insulin injections exhibited the same symptoms as individuals who had received an overdose of the hormone. The only possible explanation for this, according to Dr. Harris, was that the pancreas of these patients was responsible for the overdose of insulin, since it had not come from any outside source. The overactive gland caused a dangerously low blood sugar level in its victims. In a paper written in 1924, Dr. Harris mentioned headache as one of the symptoms of an abnormally high insulin production. Thereafter, several papers appeared in the medical literature mentioning headache as one of the symptoms of both insulin-induced and spontaneous hypoglycemia.

The first specific mention of migraine in connection with low blood sugar levels was in 1927. P. J. Cammidge wrote in the *British Medical Journal* that low blood sugar levels could be detected in persons suffering from migraine.

Some years later, McDonald Critchley and F. R. Ferguson found that migraine often began in the early morning hours, or after prolonged physical activity. They also found that starvation could bring on a migraine headache. This indicated that as the level of sugar in the blood dropped, the chances for an attack of migraine increased.

A set of papers on the same subject followed, among them the especially interesting work by P. A. Gray and H. L.

Burtness, "Hypoglycemic Headache. The authors observed a group of twenty patients with typical migraine accompanied by nausea and vomiting, and found that it was possible to avert their attacks by maintaining their blood sugar at a high level.

Oddly enough, after the publication of these early studies, we find only sporadic mention of the relationship between hypoglycemia and migraine headache in medical literature. Of particular interest, however, is a work published in 1967 by H. J. Roberts that clearly states that hypoglycemia is indeed the metabolic disorder that produces migraine.

In view of this past experience, it seems reasonable that migraine headaches could be caused by hypoglycemia, or low blood sugar, and yet it is still thought of as a mysterious disease.

3

My Search for an Answer

Many of us involved in research gravitate to a particular field because our lives have been touched personally by it. Initially I became interested in migraine for selfish reasons: I, too, was a migraine sufferer.

Among my earliest memories are Sunday outings to the park with my father when I was about six years old. Like most children, I was indulged with confectionery treats of every kind. My father would buy me a sweet and a soft drink, and then meet with his friends for long hours of talk. I barely listened to their discussions; instead, bored with adult conversation, I concentrated on feeding the squirrels and eating my treats. After a while, I would be overcome by a terrible sensation of weakness and extreme hunger, and sometimes even fainting spells. These discomforts lasted until I arrived home, and I would not feel any better until my mother gave me something to eat. In retrospect, it is clear these were not the usual childhood "junk food tummy-aches."

At school these same feelings sometimes became even more intense; only at mealtimes did I experience any relief. During these early years, I often snacked on sweets, especially chocolates and soft drinks, and no one suspected that this habit was related to my worsening health problem. Later I would realize that a clear relationship did indeed exist.

When I was twelve years old, I experienced my first migraine. One day, while walking home from school with two of my pals, my vision became impaired for no apparent reason. I could see only half of everything, a particularly frightening phenomenon that in medical terms is called *hemianopsia*. Then rapidly moving irregular patterns of luminous lines and circles, interlaced with black ones, danced before my eyes. Throbbing, hammerlike blows beat at my left temple, and the pain became so intense that my friends had to help me home. I became aware that I had also lost the feeling in my tongue, lips, the left side of my face, and the fingertips of my left hand. I was nauseated and mentally confused, and terrified that something was happening to my brain. My parents were naturally alarmed. Our family physician was summoned at once.

After a careful examination and extensive questioning, he announced, "It's nothing important, no need to worry. He's only having an attack of migraine. Of course, Rudy's is a very severe one, but it will pass in a few hours. I see this sort of thing all the time. Some are worse than others. Here, this should help." He scribbled a prescription for a popular painkiller, which, unfortunately, gave me only slight relief. The migraine had to run its course and by the following morning it was over, but from that day on I lived in constant fear of getting another attack. Fortunately, there was no recurrence for a considerable period of time, and so I allowed myself to relax somewhat.

As the years passed, my sensations of weakness and constant hunger became more intense, accompanied by fatigue, an inability to concentrate, dizziness, and a difficulty in ordering my thoughts. A second migraine caught me by surprise many years later, one evening after I had been to the movies. From then on I became a regular migraine sufferer. There were even periods when the migraines occurred daily, but at times I would be relieved of my symptoms for as long as two to three weeks. One fact, however, stood out in this pattern: I always had a migraine after viewing a movie. Logically, this led to a concern about my sight and so I consulted an ophthalmologist. I was actually disappointed when the specialist found my vision to be normal and concluded, therefore, that there was no relationship between the headaches and my eyes.

Consideration was also given to a possible psychological origin of my headaches. This was a fashionable course to take at the time, and continues to be so, particularly for illnesses that are difficult to diagnose. It did seem strange, however, that I got migraines no matter what kind of film I saw, comedy or tragedy. Only many years later did I realize the nature of the relationship between my attendance at the movies and my headaches, a relationship that had no psychological basis whatsoever. During the shows, I almost always ate my favorite type of chocolate candy, and this, as will be explained later on, was the cause of my migraine attacks at such times.

I tried to train myself to accept my handicap and live with it, but this was not easy. My recurrent migraines complicated everything I did, particularly my studies, and I wondered how I would ever manage to complete these studies and be successful in my profession.

In time I became a university professor. My work gave me a great deal of satisfaction, though it was considerably hindered at times by my attacks of migraine. Doctors who studied my case blamed everything from my gallbladder to my liver and intestines, and all of them placed me on a variety of rigorous diets. They prohibited cheese, citrus fruits, eggs, fried foods, shellfish, and innumerable other items, but to no avail.

Because the daily pressures of my job were intensified by my almost constant pain, my determination to "grin and bear it" wore thin. I became angry. There had to be a reasonable explanation for my migraines, one that could be used to give me some relief. As a scientist, I could not accept anything less. So much was being accomplished in medicine that I felt certain there was a solution somewhere for me. I decided to seek help at one of the most famous diagnostic centers in the world. After submitting me to every examination imaginable, to laboratory analyses, electroencephalograms, and X rays, the doctor in charge of my case called me to his office. He examined the results of my tests carefully and announced, "You are completely healthy. I personally feel that your problem is in your mind. I am going to give you the name of a psychiatrist and I recommend that you make an appointment." I left his office extremely irritated, because I just could not accept his diagnosis. It was difficult for me to believe that all of my very real symptoms were only in my mind.

I then went to see another well-known internist who repeated the examinations, the X rays, and the electroencephalograms. After many days of discomfort and great expense, he presented me with the same diagnosis as had the other. I was beginning to think that the doctors could be right and that perhaps my problems did actually originate in my mind. I decided to see a psychiatrist. I chose a very famous doctor with an excellent reputation to whom I recounted everything, even the most insignificant details of my life. Interminable hours, hours that could have been used productively, were wasted in his office, to say nothing of the enormous amount of money that I threw away. After many months of weekly sessions there had been no easing of my symptoms. In fact, my migraines were growing in intensity and frequency. The psychiatrist's opinion was that the treatment could only be effective over a much longer period of time, but by then both my patience and my money were gone.

After a number of years had passed with no change in my condition, I decided to look for the cause of migraine myself. I felt sure that as a chemist I had the necessary background to undertake this search, particularly since biochemistry, the science that links medicine and chemistry, was my specialty. I began to read the newest medical books available, studying all known diseases, physical and mental, whose symptoms coincided with mine. I prepared synoptic charts showing all possible relationships. My paperwork led me to the conclusion that, in addition to migraine, I also suffered from hypoglycemia, or low blood sugar. However, so little was known about this condition that the many doctors who had seen me never mentioned this to me. Then I searched textbooks for a possible treatment, but none was suggested.

One day it occurred to me to consult an old physician in the neighborhood. The advice he gave me sounded so logical that I failed to notice that he was completely wrong.

"Rudy," he said, "if you have low blood sugar, and it

appears that you do, the sugar in your bloodstream has to be increased. It is elementary to treat such cases with a diet that is rich in sugar and carbohydrates. Eat a candy bar when you feel weak or fatigued and you'll find that your energy will return."

I left his office feeling an elation that only a detective knows when he has finally solved the case. I had at last found an answer to at least part of my problem. What an easy and pleasant treatment, to boot! I not only loved sweets, but had a compulsive urge for them, so I followed my doctor's orders immediately. I stopped for a dish of strawberry ice cream on my way back to the university. My happiness was immeasurable.

I soon began to indulge my craving for sweets, which had always been uncontrollable, with great quantities of sugar. For a time, right after eating a "goody," I would feel considerably better, but unfortunately this proved to be only a temporary remedy. Soon my feelings of hunger and weakness became more pronounced, and, most regrettable of all, my migraine attacks grew worse. The treatment for hypoglycemia seemed to aggravate my migraine, as if the two diseases were mutually antagonistic. Once again pain dominated my life.

Just when my headaches became almost intolerable, I was appointed president of a leading university, a job that would require my complete and unencumbered concentration. Although I longed for this illustrious position, I wondered many times how I could possibly perform my duties competently if the migraines were to continue at their present rate.

Several weeks later, I recognized an old friend, Dr. George Villabona, in the faculty cafeteria.

"Hello, George," I called from my place in line to where

he sat. He hurried over and shook my hand vigorously. George had been a student of mine in the School of Medicine many years before. "George, what brings you to the university? You're not thinking of specializing again, are you?" I joked.

"No, I think I'm getting too old for school. I'm attending a symposium here this afternoon. Did you know that my practice is close by now? Right around the corner. Well, how have you been, Rudy?"

"Fine, fine," I said without thinking, and then quickly corrected the untruth. "Actually, I haven't been well at all. I still have my old migraine problem, and now it seems that I have hypoglycemia as well. One problem tends to complicate the other."

As we ate lunch, I explained how I had tried in vain to find an answer. My lunch consisted of a sandwich, a Coke, and a piece of cherry pie for dessert. He looked on sadly as I devoured the pie, and shook his head.

"Rudy, you are eating all the wrong kinds of food for someone who has hypoglycemia," he said. "Have you ever had a glucose tolerance test performed to be sure that you do have low blood sugar?"

I shook my head.

"You really should have one done to be absolutely sure, but from the symptoms you've described, it sounds as if you do.* Of course, you're familiar with the test, aren't you? It's used mainly to diagnose diabetes." I had known this test at one time, but to refresh my memory he drew crude diagrams on a couple of paper napkins as he spoke.

"Now," he began, "if you give a normal individual, after

---

*Shortly after my meeting with Dr. George Villabona, a glucose tolerance test was performed on me and it proved conclusively that I suffered from low blood sugar.

he has fasted overnight, one hundred grams of glucose, and then take blood samples every hour and analyze for sugar, you will get a pattern something like this [see Figure 1]. Can you see that after about three hours the blood sugar approaches the normal fasting range once again? This range is usually somewhere between seventy and ninety milligrams per one hundred milliliters of blood."

"Yes, yes," I said rather impatiently, since now I remembered and needed no further elaboration to understand his lesson. He obviously enjoyed lecturing his old teacher, however, and would not be stopped.

"A person who is a diabetic does not produce enough insulin to metabolize the sugar in his blood," Dr. Villabona continued. "His curve would probably look something like this [see Figure 2]. Notice that a diabetic's fasting blood sugar is higher than that of a normal individual. One hour after ingesting the sugar solution, it usually has increased to about one hundred eighty or more, and five hours after ingesting, it is still higher than the fasting level." He looked satisfied and took just a moment to improve on his drawings. "Now you understand why diabetics must have insulin injections to reduce their blood sugar to normal.

"And now," he said, "let us go to your case.

"The pancreas of a diabetic does not produce enough insulin, but yours manufactures too much. How delicately balanced the body must be to perform just right." He pondered the profundity of this, and, I must admit, so did I.

"Anyway," he continued, "if we performed a glucose tolerance test on you, it would approximate this kind of curve— if you are indeed a hypoglycemic [see Figure 3]. After one hour your blood sugar would probably be only in the range of one hundred twenty. Compare this with the values for the normal and the diabetic individuals. Notice how low

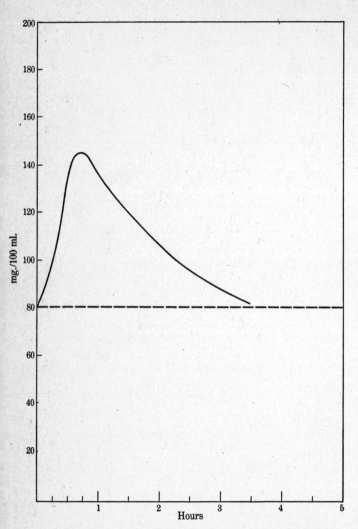

Figure 1. *Variation of the concentration of glucose in the blood of a normal individual after ingesting 100 grams of glucose.*

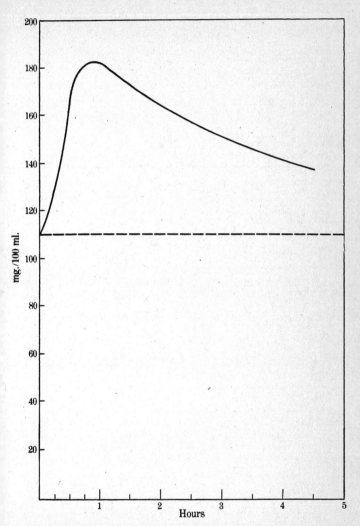

Figure 2. Variation of the concentration of glucose in the blood of a diabetic individual after ingesting 100 grams of glucose.

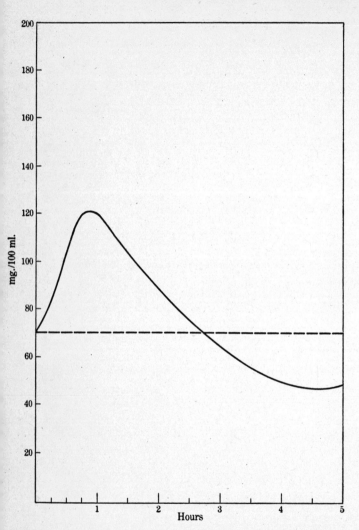

Figure 3. *Variation of the concentration of glucose in the blood of a hypoglycemic individual after ingesting 100 grams of glucose.*

your blood sugar in all likelihood would be after five hours, much lower than even your fasting value. Your body produces too much insulin and this uses up not only the sugar given in the test, but part of the sugar normally contained in the blood as well. Can you imagine now what happens when you eat the kind of food you are eating?

"Your body is already producing too much insulin; when you eat sugar, it is stimulated to produce even more. Think of it as a circle. You eat sugar, and your pancreas overresponds with an excess of insulin. This in turn uses up not only the sugar you have eaten, but also part of your blood sugar; and this makes you hungry. You then satisfy this hunger by eating again, probably something sweet, and the cycle begins again. You see then that the sugar you eat is responsible for your low blood sugar or hypoglycemia. Therefore, the answer for you is simply do without sugar. Moreover, you may find it interesting that I read somewhere that migraine headache is brought on by hypoglycemia."

Dr. Villabona was really well informed. None of the many doctors who studied my case had ever referred to this. He actually motivated me to initiate the research that ultimately gave me the answer to the question of what causes migraine headache and how it can be relieved.

I couldn't sleep that night, not because of migraine but because of the excitement the day's talk had generated in me. My brain raced over all the new and powerful ideas that had been hypothesized by my old friend. It all began to fall into place. I had felt sick as a boy after eating treats made with sugar. Since my trips to the movies always included candy, they too helped to bring on my attacks. The right path had finally been opened up to me. My family doctor, like so many others, had been mistaken in his treatment for low blood sugar.

By morning, I had made a decision to give up sugar completely, and I did so. The results were astounding. In a few days, the migraine attacks decreased in frequency and intensity, and all of my other symptoms—weakness, hunger, fatigue, dizziness, lack of concentration, and the inability to coordinate my thoughts—also improved considerably.

A new life began for me after I completely eliminated sugar from my diet, though my recovery was not total. Since Dr. Villabona had mentioned a relationship between migraine and hypoglycemia, I once again searched the medical literature to see if I could further improve my condition. I reviewed the most up-to-date medical texts and found that none of them alluded to such a relationship. Although I found a few scientific papers, most of them written in the thirties, that suggested that hypoglycemia could be the triggering agent in an attack of migraine, they were never considered serious enough to be included in medical textbooks.*

I then decided to investigate for myself and determine if hypoglycemia was the precipitating factor of migraine in predisposed individuals. I measured blood sugar levels before, during, and after migraine attacks. I also investigated the effects of various carbohydrates on the concentration of sugar in the blood, as well as their ability to stimulate the pancreas to produce insulin. The latter factor was determined by measuring the insulin concentration in the blood after the ingestion of several common carbohydrates. These experiments were conducted on healthy subjects as well as on migraine sufferers. Finally, I compared the reaction of the pancreas to both refined sugar and the unprocessed carbohydrates found in natural foods. My research proved that only refined sugar stimulated the pancreas of predis-

---

*These papers are referred to in the Bibliography.

posed individuals to produce too much insulin. The unprocessed carbohydrates found in natural foods did not have a similar effect.*

My research began to shed more and more light on the causes of migraine. I then initiated a treatment for myself that eliminated all of my symptoms, without exception.

*See references under Low in the Bibliography.

4

Sweet Sorrow

Sugarcane, which contains an average of 17 percent sugar, has been known to man since ancient times. Although some authors contend that India is the home of the grassy reed *Saccharum officinarum*, most agree, in light of exhaustive botanical studies, that it probably originated somewhere around 8000 B.C. in New Guinea, where it was grown domestically for chewing. From there its cultivation moved in a southeasterly course to the Solomon Islands, the New Hebrides, and New Caledonia. From about 6000 B.C. onward, the cane traveled west to the Philippines, Indonesia, and finally to northern India, where we find the earliest record of the plant. In the *Atharva-Veda*, the last part of the ancient sacred books of the Hindus, there is a reference to sugar. The *Atharva-Veda* dates back to about 1000 B.C. and consists of a collection of hymns and prayers. It is in these books that we find the passage: "I have crowned thee with a shooting sugarcane, so thou shalt not be adverse to me."

In Sanskrit, the ancient language of India, the word for sugar is *sarkara* or *sakkara*, which means "sand" or "gravel." This later became *sukkar* in Arabic, *sucre* in French, *sakkharon* in Greek, *azúcar* in Spanish, and *sugar* in English. From India, the cultivation of cane and a process for extracting its sweet juice spread to Persia, Arabia, and Egypt.

Although there is no mention of sugar in ancient Egyptian or Chinese writings, we do find its use hinted at in the Bible. The following passage can be found in Jeremiah 6:20:

> To what purpose cometh there to me incense from Sheba, and the sweet cane from a far country? Your burnt offerings are not acceptable nor your sacrifices sweet unto me.

And in Isaiah 43:24 we find:

> Thou hast bought me no sweet cane with money, neither hast thou filled me with the fat of thy sacrifices; but thou hast made me to serve with thy sins, thou hast wearied me with thine iniquities.

In 325 B.C., an officer in the invading army of Alexander the Great in India spoke of a plant that produced "honey without the aid of bees." The campaigns of Alexander the Great are thus credited with the spread of sugarcane to many parts of Europe. Here it became an expensive treasure and, because of its scarcity, a gift only for kings and queens and the very rich. Before the advent of sugar, man satisfied his lust for sweets by eating fruit and honey, but when he discovered the existence of sugarcane he soon became tired of nature's more abundant treats and sought to place the priceless cane within his reach.

Just exactly where sugar making had its beginnings is disputed by the experts. Some insist that there is no earlier evidence of the process than that which began in Persia around 500 A.D., while other authors credit India with initiating the technology, dating it from the fourth to the sixth century. In ancient sugar processing, the cane was cut into small pieces and the juice extracted by crushing these with heavy weights. The liquid was then boiled, creating a solid material that looked like gravel (hence the Sanskrit name, *sarkara*) as the end product. This sugar was not like the white crystals that we know today. Coarse and brown in color, it still contained many of its natural components. As the refining process became more sophisticated, more of sugar's proteins, vitamins, and minerals were removed.

The enormous amount of world travel and trade that occurred during the seventh, eighth, and ninth centuries was responsible for the introduction of sugar refining to other geographical areas. The Arabs and the Egyptians learned to purify this gravel-like material, leading to the birth of the sweetmeat or "goody" made with processed sugar. The Egyptians also initiated the use of lime in the refining process, allowing the soluble nonsugar components to separate out when the cane juice was heated.

By the eighth century, sugarcane had been taken to Arabic Spain and southern France, where it developed into a prosperous industry. In short supply and thus very expensive, sugar was used in Europe mainly for medicinal purposes; it was used in many medieval formulas, in particular as a sedative. When sugar was first introduced into Great Britain, its price was approximately twenty-five American dollars per pound—the salary of an average worker for one year.

Sugarcane was brought to the West Indies early in the sixteenth century, and the natives found that the plant thrived in their tropical islands. Among the English colonists who came to America in the seventeenth century, there were those who settled on the Caribbean islands of St. Christopher, Barbados, Nevis, Montserrat, and Antigua. Although tobacco was the crop tried first by the settlers in these regions, as it was on the mainland, they soon learned how much more profitable it was to grow and process sugarcane. Before sugar cultivation commenced in the West Indies, England was largely dependent on the regions of the Mediterranean for its sparse supply. The southern European climate, however, was too cool in the winter and not humid enough for maximum sugar production. In the tropical West Indies, it could be grown practically year round. In a relatively short time the islanders became quite adept at the large-scale manufacturing of sugar; and since this meant huge profits for the planter, they utilized every available acre for the cultivation of cane. Thus food and lumber became scarce, and the islanders were forced to import these necessities so that they could continue to work full speed at sugar production. Many people probably think slavery in the New World originated on the large tobacco plantations of the Carolinas and Virginia in the colonial United States. In fact, slavery was adopted relatively late on the American mainland. It was the planter class of the West Indies who found that it was most profitable to engage large numbers of black slaves in the fast-growing sugar industry.

Prior to the introduction of slavery, the plantation owners had depended on the natives and on indentured labor to keep their farms and sugar mills operating. The whites who were indentured were usually men, and sometimes women, who had been convicted of a crime and as punishment were bound to work for the planter who had bought their services. The term of bondage was usually three or four years, during which they received from their master food, clothing, and shelter while in his employment, freedom once their term of indenture had expired, and paid passage back to their homeland when they were freed. An African slave, on the other hand, cost his owner only the initial price of fifteen to twenty-five pounds, could be fed and clothed cheaply, and worked for his entire life.

Sugar growing and refining, then, played an enormous role in the enslavement and exploitation of huge numbers of African men, women, and children. The West Indies are today about 95 percent black. England tried, in the eighteenth and nineteenth centuries, to put an end to slavery in its West Indian islands, but the profits from the number-one commodity on the European market were just too large and the demand for sugar too urgent to allow this. The Act for the Abolishment of Slavery was finally passed on August 1, 1834, but by then hundreds of thousands of Africans had been transported from their homeland and forced to live (probably not too long) without freedom in a foreign land. And man's lust for sugar persisted.

The sugar beet, like other beets a fleshy rooted plant of the goosefoot family, is reported by some scholars to have been eaten by the laborers who built the pyramid for the Egyptian pharaoh Cheops, who lived about 3000 B.C. Indeed, early writers made references to the beet root, and Hippocrates noted that the plant's leaves had healing properties when applied to wounds. *Beta vulgaris*, the sugar beet, grows best in temperate climates, unlike the sugarcane plant, which thrives in the tropics. In 1747 Andreas Marggraf, a German chemist, proved that sucrose was stored in the usually yellowish-white root of the beet and that this precious commodity could be extracted from it. Just over half a century later, one of Marggraf's pupils, Franz C.

Achard, was successful in obtaining large quantities of sugar from beets, which contain about 14 percent sugar. In 1812 Benjamin Delessert found a way to process this sugar into an acceptable commercial product. Not until after the emancipation of the black slaves in the West Indies was the sugar-beet industry in Europe able to compete successfully with tropical sugars. Principal producers today are Germany, France, and Russia. In the United States the production of sugar from beets in thousand metric tons was 5,900 in 1913. In 1983 this figure was only 2,700.

Sugar refining today has become a highly technical and efficient industry, dedicated to the production of the whitest and purest crystals possible. Purity is a commandment in itself for the sugar czars. Any of nature's nutrients, including precious proteins, vitamins, and minerals, that might have been present in the sugarcane or sugar beet plant are lost in the process of refinement. This is where the money is: in purity.

In the modern technology of sugar refining the beets are cut into small pieces and placed in large containers with hot water to dissolve the sugar. If sugarcane is used, it is first cut into chips and the juice is pressed out by passing them through a mill. The sugar solution in the first case or the juice in the second case is filtered to remove suspended impurities, and lime is then added to neutralize the acidity of the juice, to precipitate out the dissolved nonsugar components, and to decolorize the juice. The mixture is then heated and allowed to settle in large tanks called clarifiers. Sometimes sulfur dioxide is used to neutralize the excess lime and to help further decolorize the juice. Once clarification is completed, the juice is filtered and concentrated by vacuum boiling until sugar crystallizes out. The crystals are separated from the liquid by centrifugation. The remaining liquid, called molasses, is again boiled and then separated into a second raw sugar and second molasses; and then the process is repeated a third time. The raw sugar is shipped to a refinery, where it is dissolved in hot water to be again decolorized and filtered. The color of the liquid at this stage is somewhere between straw yellow and brown. It is percolated through special chemical products that absorb the color-producing ingredients and yield a completely clear fluid. This liquid is once again concentrated, crystallized, centrifuged, and dried. Is it any wonder that pure sucrose is all that remains of the original product? The human body has no need whatsoever for pure sugar, and in fact, as you shall see, is actually harmed by it. The medical profession is already aware of the detrimental effects of refined sugar on the human body; let us hope that this book will challenge it also to accept the truth about sugar's role in migraine.

According to A. C. Barnes, at least twenty million acres of the earth's land surface are devoted to the growing of sugarcane, and the quantity harvested and processed each year amounts to 320 million long tons. In 1974 the world's production of sugar in thousand metric tons was 76,397 and by 1981 it had risen to 91,932. This trend has been steady throughout sugar's long history. Affluence seems to determine just how much sugar and how many products made with it an individual consumes. Wealth brings with it more conveniences, more television sets, more leisure time and vacations, more entertaining and dining out, and—more drinks and snacks loaded with refined sugar. The total sugar consumption in the United States alone in 1983 was 9,400 thousand metric tons. An average American puts over seventy pounds of sugar annually into his or her body—almost one and one half pounds per week! It's hard to believe, isn't it? You're saying to yourself, "No! I don't eat that much sugar. It's impossible." It may appear incredible, but it is far from impossible. I am not saying that the average consumer gobbles up one five-pound bag after another. This would be repulsive to even the greediest addict. Sugar, however, is masked in such delightful favorites as cakes, candies, caramels, canned fruits, chocolates, cookies, custards, dried fruits, fruit juices, fruit-flavored yogurts, jams, soft drinks, and sweet liqueurs and wines. Even more alarming, there are large amounts of sugar in less obvious places, including baby foods, canned vegetables, cereals, frozen dinners, and sauces and garnishes. Did you know that a twelve-ounce can of soft drink can have as much as 20 grams of sugar in it, and that a jelly doughnut may yield 30 grams? Thirty grams of sugar is equivalent to approximately six teaspoonsful. The manufacturers know what we like and what we'll buy, so they include sucrose in almost every conceivable food product on the market today. Our sugar habit has a reputable and faithful supplier—a world economy dedicated to the profit motive. Many people openly confess that they are compulsive sugar eaters. I have seen people take a small cup, fill it three-quarters full with tea, add milk, and then dump in four teaspoonsful of sugar. What a dangerous and, to my way of thinking, unpalatable concoction!

Diabetes

We have already seen the hazards for the hypoglycemic of indulging in sugar, an issue that will be discussed in detail later in this book. The opposite of hypoglycemia, or low blood sugar, is hyperglycemia, or high blood sugar. It is usually the result of the failure of the pancreas to produce enough insulin, although in some instances the body is not able to utilize the insulin. High blood sugar generates many unpleasant and dangerous symptoms that constitute the

disease known as diabetes. This means that both hypoglycemia and its opposite, hyperglycemia, or diabetes, are
usually the result of a malfunctioning of the insulin-producing
cells in the pancreas. If sugar affects one disorder, shouldn't
it have some influence on the other also? We know that once
a person has contracted diabetes, he must carefully watch
his intake of refined sugars, since his insulin is in short
supply and cannot handle the extra burden of large amounts
of sugar. Can a person who has a family tendency to diabetes
control his fate in any way? The answer is an emphatic yes.
If an individual's pancreas malfunctions, it has most likely
been abused in some way. True, heredity plays its part in
the development of the disease, but so does the constant
year-in, year-out bombardment of the insulin-producing cells
with large quantities of almost 100 percent pure sugar. The
pancreas of such a person can take only so much. It strug-
gles for years to balance the body's metabolism by a constant outpouring of insulin. Alas, it can do this no longer,
having worn itself out.

There is a definite relationship between an individual's
sugar intake and the development of diabetes. In adults,
an overweight condition of the body usually precedes the
onset of the disease. According to a report of diabetics by
Louis I. Dublin, the males in the study group who were 25
percent or more overweight had a death rate from diabetes
thirteen times higher than those who were underweight.
Death rates from diabetes are generally up in the white
population of western Europe and the British Common-
wealth, where sugar consumption is high, and low in eastern
and southern Europe and the Orient, where less sugar is
consumed. From the *Statistical Abstract of the United States*
for 1984 and from previous editions of the same work we
find that the per capita consumption of sugar rose from 97.6
pounds annually in 1960 to over 100 pounds in 1970 and then

Table 1. Death Rates from Diabetes in the United States (per 100,000 population)

1960	16.7
1965	17.1
1970	18.9
1975	16.4
1980	15.4
1981	15.1

began to decrease, until it was 71 pounds in 1983. This fortunate trend was probably influenced by the many publications of the last years pointing out the health-threatening effect of refined sugar.

The same statistical source also shows that death rates from diabetes in the United States increased to a maximum of 18.9 per 100,000 population in 1970 and then began to decrease (see Table 1).

The fact that the death rates from diabetes in the United States increased when the per capita consumption of sugar was increasing and then began to decrease when the consumption of sugar was decreasing can hardly be considered a simple coincidence. Rather, it indicates an actual relationship between sugar consumption and death rates from diabetes.

Heart Disease

The argument over the cause of cardiovascular disease has continued for many years. However, one predominant factor noted in studies is that cardiovascular disease is far more prevalent in affluent societies than in underdeveloped countries. Our number-one killer walks hand in hand with a sedentary life, excessive cigarette smoking, and overeating. The chances of death from cardiovascular disease increase with the number of pounds that an individual carries around. A study reported by Louis I. Dublin shows that the mortality from cardiovascular disease among males 20 percent overweight is 25 percent higher than for those maintaining a normal weight. For males who are 30 percent overweight, the death rate is 42 percent higher than that of individuals of average weight. Women who are 20 percent overweight show a mortality rate from cardiovascular disease 20 percent higher than that for women of normal weight, and for those 30 percent overweight it is 30 percent higher.

The fastest way to increase your weight is to indulge yourself with large quantities of goods that are high in sugar. Fatty foods do contribute to obesity to a certain degree, but the main culprit is sugar. Food with a high fat content, such as pork, does have some redeeming qualities to justify its consumption—namely, it is a protein food that also contains many essential vitamins and minerals. Refined sucrose, however, cannot boast of even this, and in addition, the sugar not used for the body's immediate needs or for storage is converted by the liver to fat. The bathroom scale then broadcasts the sad news.

Atherosclerosis is a disease in which small masses, called *atheromas*, develop in the arterial walls. These masses undergo a series of changes that can lead to hardening of the arteries and eventually to a blockage in the vessel. The atheromas are actually localized thickenings in the blood vessel walls consisting of fatty material; eventually they result in the formation of scar tissue on the inside of the vessel wall.

There has been much talk about cholesterol levels in relation to atherosclerosis, since in the disease this compound is present with the lipid material in the atheromas. A normal individual eats about 0.3 grams of cholesterol daily. The body itself synthesizes an additional 1.5 to 2.0 grams of cholesterol each day. Cholesterol is, in fact, needed by the body in the synthesis of the steroid hormones, which control the secondary sex characteristics, the reproductive cycle, and the growth and development of the accessory reproductive organs. If a person were to eat no cholesterol whatsoever for one day, his body would still manufacture it on its own (from 1.5 to 2.0 grams). If he were to eat a large amount of a food that is high in cholesterol—for instance, eggs—his body would adjust to the situation by simply synthesizing the smaller amount. So you see, the cholesterol question still needs much study.

Many people who are so very careful about their cholesterol intake, using egg and cheese substitutes, the margarine with the highest degree of unsaturation, skim milk or no milk at all, still continue to eat all of the refined sugar they want. Their weight goes up, they feel bad, and they become good risks for cardiovascular disease. I am not completely discarding the theory that cholesterol plays some part in the development of atherosclerosis; however, I do question the importance given to its role.

Diseases of the Digestive Tract

About thirteen million Americans suffer from some disease of the digestive tract, and gastric disorders are the number-one reason for hospitalization in the United States today. These statistics emphasize the ill effects of sugar on the digestive organs because the United States, as a very wealthy nation, is one of the highest per capita consumers of sugar in the world. A very significant pattern is thus developing linking sugar to the incidence of many of our modern diseases.

Refined sugar has a great capacity to irritate the lining of the digestive organs, causing an increase in the acidity there and an excessive secretion of gastric juices. If you wonder why you can't eat without suffering the discomforts of chronic heartburn, ask yourself what kinds of foods you are eating. Do you eat nothing more than a doughnut or other sweet bun for breakfast and drink a soft drink or two with lunch? Are you constantly munching on cookies or candy bars? Try doing without sugar for a week or so and watch the improvement.

In areas of the stomach and the adjacent small intestine that are exposed regularly to excess acid and gastric juices, a far more serious problem may be developing. The mucous membrane of these essential digestive organs can become ulcerated; if the damage extends deeply enough into the wall of the stomach or the small intestine, you have, respectively, a gastric or a duodenal ulcer. Then, of course, you will be forced to watch what you eat. Doesn't it make more sense to do the watching before the trouble begins? In the Western world, gastric ulcer is a common disease found in 10 percent of all men, and 2 percent of all women, over the age of fifty. Duodenal ulcer is also more common in men than in women and has its onset early in life, usually appearing before the age of twenty-five.

Tooth Decay

Dentists have been warning us for years to keep our children away from treats made with refined sugar so that they may have healthier teeth. However, according to the U.S. Department of Health, Education and Welfare, of every one hundred Americans, fewer than five go through life without tooth decay. By the time an average child is old enough to go to school, he already has three decayed teeth. Children over fourteen have an average of eleven cavities, and by the time they reach middle age, two out of three people will have serious problems. Why haven't we listened to our dentists? We haven't listened because we are programmed to seek our pleasure before our health, no matter what the price. Oh, sure, we'll brush more, have frequent checkups, use our dental floss, but we won't interfere with the short-lived happiness that we derive from eating sweets.

Tooth decay is caused by plaque, a sticky, practically invisible substance that adheres to the teeth. It is made up of decomposed food particles and millions of living bacteria. Plaque is held on to the teeth by a substance called dextran, which is composed mostly of sugars. When we eat food containing refined sugars, the bacteria in the plaque produce acids that dissolve the enamel of the tooth, and decay begins. When the plaque is not removed, it becomes calcified and can lead to periodontal disease, and eventually to the loss of teeth.

We have heard all of this before, and yet we continue to reward ourselves—and much worse, our children—with the dubious prize of treats made with sugar.

5

Sugar and Your Aching Head

Sugars and starch belong to a large group of compounds, found abundantly in nature, known as carbohydrates, which are composed of carbon, hydrogen, and oxygen, the last two in the same proportion as in water. These compounds are always ingredients of natural products that also contain many other compounds. For instance, a fruit usually contains less than 20 percent of sugars and the balance—that is, over 80 percent—is a blend of other compounds. Vegetables sometimes contain a high percentage of starch, but in addition they contain many other compounds.

The simplest of these carbohydrates, called *monosaccharides*, are substances that cannot be broken down any further into simpler sugars in the digestive process; therefore they are also known as simple sugars. Three of the most important monosaccharides, from both the nutritive and the physiological points of view, are glucose, fructose, and galactose. Glucose, which is also known by the name dextrose, is found in varying amounts in different fruits and in small quantities in human blood. When a glucose tolerance test is performed on an individual to determine the amount of sugar in his blood, it is the monosaccharide glucose that is actually measured. Glucose is the chief form in which the living body utilizes sugar. Fructose, also called "fruit sugar," is found in most fruits, and galactose is found combined with glucose in the disaccharide lactose, or "milk sugar."

Disaccharides are compounds composed of two simple sugars linked by a chemical bond. Sucrose, a disaccharide found in many fruits and plants, is the carbohydrate that is extracted in great quantities from sugarcane and sugar beets for commercial use. The white crystals that you spoon into your coffee several times a day are pure sucrose, the sugar from the cane and beet plants, stripped of its proteins, vitamins, and minerals. Sucrose is composed equally of the two simple sugars, glucose and fructose. Another disaccharide of interest is maltose, formed in germinating grains and present in large quantities in corn syrup and beer. Disaccharides are easily converted into monosaccharides and are therefore sometimes referred to, although improperly, as simple sugars.

Some carbohydrates are composed of great chains of simple sugars "hooked" together to form one enormous molecule. They are called *polysaccharides*, or complex carbohydrates; starch, the storage form of carbohydrate in plants, is one of the most important of these. Another polysaccharide is glycogen, or animal starch, the storage form of carbohydrate in the animal body.

In order to avoid any confusion in the following pages it is necessary to know that when the term *natural sugar* is used in the text, reference is made to the complete natural product containing it, such as a fruit or fruit juice, while *refined sugar* or *pure sugar* means the pure chemical compound from which all other components provided by nature have been removed. The term *processed sugar* means the same, but it will not be used in the text.

On the other hand, when *natural carbohydrate* is used, reference is usually made to a natural product containing a complex carbohydrate, such as potatoes, wheat, or rice, although natural carbohydrate can obviously also refer to a natural fruit. Finally, if a natural product containing a complex carbohydrate is processed, some, but by no means all, of the other components are removed. This is the case with white wheat flour, which still contains many of its natural components and is therefore not harmful for the hypoglycemic. Pure starch would be as harmful as pure sugar, but it is never found as an ingredient of foods; it does indeed exist, but only as a laboratory curiosity.

All carbohydrates, regardless of size, are broken down by the digestive system and utilized by the body, chiefly in the form of glucose. By the time a carbohydrate reaches the small intestine, where food is absorbed into the bloodstream, it has already been metabolized into its simplest characteristic fragments.

Each molecule of glucose passes through the intestinal wall into the bloodstream, and soon reaches the liver. Here part of the glucose is converted into "stored sugar," or glycogen, by the action of an enzyme. This glycogen remains stored in the liver and also in the muscles until the body has a need for it. The greater part of the glucose continues to circulate through the body, producing a temporary hyperglycemia, or increased sugar concentration in the blood.

To understand what happens to this glucose in its tour through the body, it is necessary to understand a bit about the endocrine glands. These glands are a group of organs that secrete, directly into the bloodstream, a variety of chemical substances called hormones. Each of the endocrine glands performs specific functions, although the activities of one usually influence those of the others. The endocrine glands are interconnected through the bloodstream, and the hormones they secrete regulate—speed up or slow down and, above all, coordinate—all functions of the body. There are many endocrines, but two especially concern the migraine patient: the adrenals and the pancreas.

The two adrenal glands are located above the kidneys. Each consists of two parts, the medulla and the cortex, like a nut and its shell. The cortex of the adrenals produces no fewer than thirty-two hormones, and it is now considered by some to be of even greater importance than the pituitary, or "master" gland. The secretions of the adrenal cortex control the chemical processes that convert food into the substances responsible for making the body grow, change, and function properly. The adrenal medulla secretes a group of hormones called the *catecholamines*, among which epinephrine, also known as adrenaline, is the most important. Other catecholamines are noradrenaline or norepinephrine and dopamine. If the blood sugar should fall below normal for any reason, the adrenals come to the rescue by releasing adrenaline and the other catecholamines. These hormones, in turn, convert the "stored sugar" in the liver into glucose once again.

The pancreas is a long, narrow gland located deep in the abdominal cavity. Its extreme right end is directly connected to the small intestine, into which the pancreatic juice, needed for proper digestion, passes. In addition, the pancreas produces two hormones, insulin and glucagon. While the function of glucagon is to increase the amount of glucose in the blood, insulin has the ability to decrease it, a fact that has become common knowledge, since diabetics use insulin expressly for this purpose.

When the blood containing the newly digested sugar passes through the pancreas, the pancreas's specialized cells release insulin to permit metabolism of the carbohydrate to take place. The healthy pancreas does not produce insulin when the glucose concentration is within normal limits, (generally between 70 and 90 milligrams per 100 milliliters of blood). However, when the sugar in the blood increases, the extra glucose stimulates the pancreas to release insulin in order to offset the increment.

Just how does insulin accomplish this? It performs essentially four tasks:

1. It helps the liver to convert sugar into glycogen for storage.
2. It helps the muscles, in the same way, to transform glucose into glycogen, which is held in reserve for the times when the body needs it.
3. It prevents the reverse phenomenon, that is, the conversion of glycogen into glucose.
4. It activates the oxidation of glucose within the cells in order to provide energy, a process in which the sugar is broken down into water and carbon dioxide.

The human body is run by an infinitely complex system of delicately balanced and interrelated chemical reactions. Each small reaction is responsible in part for the total healthy functioning of a human being. Sugar metabolism involves a series of biochemical interreactions that must be in perfect balance for good health. Sometimes this equilibrium in the body is upset. If one of these tiny chemical reactions is an overresponse or is too small, the human body is no longer in perfect health. A malfunction will develop in the area for which this reaction is responsible. For example, an underactive thyroid gland can cause an increase in weight; if it is overactive, the symptoms include loss of weight and nervousness. Underactivity of the pituitary results in a condition known as infantilism, a failure of the body to attain maturity; overactivity of this gland results in a progressive enlargement of hands, feet, and face—or in medical terms, acromegaly. Underactivity of the adrenal glands often results in Addison's disease, while overactivity can cause accentuated masculine characteristics to develop in either sex.

When an underactive pancreas secretes insufficient insulin for the metabolism of sugar, diabetes results. Diabetics have an excess of glucose in their blood and must be given injections of insulin in order to correct this abnormality. The opposite condition—known as hyperinsulinism—though less well known, is caused by a pancreas that produces too much insulin. The excess of insulin consumes a larger amount of glucose than necessary, generating a disorder called hypoglycemia, or low blood sugar. Although an overactive pancreas, or hyperinsulinism, is the most frequent cause of hypoglycemia, this disorder may also be due to other causes, such as certain diseases of the liver or irregularities of the thyroid and pituitary glands.

It is clear then that one does not suffer from hypoglycemia because one does not eat enough sugar, but because of an overactive pancreas that is producing too much insulin. When a hypoglycemic individual eats sugar, his pancreas is stimulated to secrete insulin; however, because of the abnormality in the mechanism of his gland, the insulin that is produced will be in excess of what is actually needed. This overabundance of insulin metabolizes not only the newly ingested sugar but also some of the glucose that was already present in his bloodstream. The result is a state of low blood sugar and its distressing symptoms, among which can be a migraine headache.

After participating in a very strenuous physical activity, a healthy person feels tired; his energy has been drained. If he rests, however, his strength will return in time. What has actually happened? The strenuous activity has burned up a great portion of the immediately available glucose— needed to satisfy the extraordinary demands that were made on the body. Then, without the intake of additional nourishment, the blood sugar level returns to normal—the "stored sugar" having been utilized to bring about the balance. The catecholamines, particularly adrenaline, are insulin opponents. Insulin decreases the blood sugar if it is too high; the catecholamines can, if the need arises, cause the blood sugar to increase, by allowing the conversion of glycogen into glucose (see Figure 4). Thus the healthy body has a unique system of checks and balances.

In a hypoglycemic person this system does not work. To perform a task requiring a great deal of energy, much of the individual's blood glucose is also used. But in this case, the glucose circulating in the body is not automatically restored to a normal level. Now what has happened? In response to a low blood sugar, the antagonist catecholamines have brought about the conversion of glycogen into glucose. Unlike the process in a healthy individual, in the hypoglycemic the new glucose stimulates the pancreas to secrete more insulin—which once again lowers the blood sugar to a dangerous level. The pancreas of the hypoglycemic is extremely sensitive to even small quantities of pure glucose, no matter what the source. It overreacts to glucose with a secretion of insulin too large to maintain an equilibrium in the body, and the patient suffers the symptoms of hypoglycemia, perhaps including a migraine.

Furthermore, the pancreas of individuals suffering from low blood sugar is frequently so overactive that it not only produces large amounts of insulin under the stimulation of

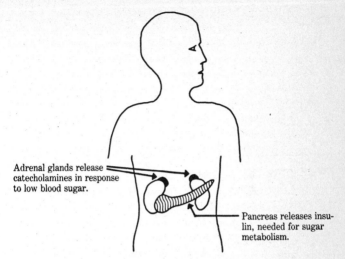

Adrenal glands release catecholamines in response to low blood sugar.

Pancreas releases insulin, needed for sugar metabolism.

Figure 4. Diagram showing the release by the pancreas of insulin, which converts part of blood sugar into glycogen or "stored sugar" in the liver and muscles, and the release by the adrenal glands of catecholamines, which convert the glycogen again into blood sugar.

sugar, but even *without* this incitement it secretes a quantity of the hormone sufficient to reduce the blood sugar level below normal. This phenomenon occurs most often two to three hours after a meal. Obviously, sugar cannot be given to a hypoglycemic at this point to raise his blood sugar, since this would only further stimulate his abnormally active pancreas to produce even more insulin. True, there would be a momentary increase in the blood glucose level; however, in a short time it would drop to an even lower value than that with which the patient started. What then is he to do? The answer is very simple. He must eat every two to three hours, and he must eat foods that are rich in protein and natural carbohydrates, in other words, foods that will not have a stimulating effect on his pancreas. It is from these sources that a hypoglycemic's body will be provided with the necessary glucose to raise his blood sugar to a normal level.

"Fine," you may say, "I understand all of this, but why does my head hurt? How does low blood sugar trigger an attack of migraine?"

We have already seen that insulin is released when an individual ingests sugar, so that the sugar can be metabolized. In a hypoglycemic, this insulin response is too great, leaving too little glucose in the blood. Adrenaline and the other catecholamines are then secreted in an attempt to rectify the situation, as they facilitate the conversion of glycogen into glucose.

Adrenaline is familiar as the body chemical released in times of great stress. Besides the important role it plays in metabolism, it has the ability to reduce the caliber of the blood vessels, thus forcing the blood to circulate with greater force. In addition, it raises the body temperature and dilates the air ducts, so that the lungs can receive additional oxygen more rapidly. Of particular interest to the migraine sufferer is that adrenaline is also acting as a powerful vasoconstrictor. This is the key to unraveling the mystery of migraine.

Sugar initiates the production of insulin by the pancreas. If the pancreas malfunctions and releases more insulin than is actually needed, reducing the blood sugar level below normal, the adrenal glands will respond in kind. At the same time that excessive adrenaline attempts to balance the body's metabolism, its other effects are also magnified, especially the reduction of the diameter of the blood vessels, which initiates the migraine attack. The visual disturbances that occur just prior to the onset of the pain can be directly correlated with this reduction of the diameter of the blood vessels. By observing the arterioles—the small terminal twigs of the arteries—in the whites of the eyes at the beginning of a migraine, one can actually see this happening. The arteriole's strong muscular wall is capable of completely closing the passageway, or of permitting it to expand to several times its normal size.

The body has a strong need to maintain its state of equilibrium. Thus, after a period of time, the vasoconstriction is followed by its opposite, a vasodilation, or expansion of the diameter of the blood vessels. Vasodilation is the result of still another set of chemical reactions that are a response to the action of adrenaline and the other catecholamines. Prostaglandins that act as strong vasodilators are produced by the body in this stage. By observing the arterioles in

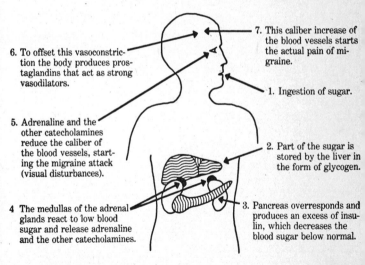

6. To offset this vasoconstriction the body produces prostaglandins that act as strong vasodilators.

7. This caliber increase of the blood vessels starts the actual pain of migraine.

1. Ingestion of sugar.

5. Adrenaline and the other catecholamines reduce the caliber of the blood vessels, starting the migraine attack (visual disturbances).

2. Part of the sugar is stored by the liver in the form of glycogen.

4 The medullas of the adrenal glands react to low blood sugar and release adrenaline and the other catecholamines.

3. Pancreas overresponds and produces an excess of insulin, which decreases the blood sugar below normal.

Figure 5. *Diagram showing how the intake of sugar can lead to the pain of migraine in hypoglycemic individuals who are predisposed to the disease.*

the eye, we can actually see, in case after case, that the pain of a migraine begins when the vessels expand.

In my original tests to confirm this fact, I injected several of my volunteer patients, including myself, with one milligram of adrenaline. In every instance, this amount of adrenaline injected into an individual predisposed to migraine precipitated an attack. However, when I injected volunteers who did not suffer from migraine with up to twice this amount of adrenaline, an attack was never generated. It appears, then, that one must both have the predisposition for the disease and experience the initiating factors for an attack to occur.

For a summary of how the intake of sugar can lead to the pain of migraine see Figure 5 (on page 51).

6

Characteristic Insulin Production in the Migraine Patient

Robert Sherman, a former chemistry student of mine, was bright and unusually gifted in the sciences. I was convinced that he had the potential for a brilliant career in chemistry, since he possessed a rare knack for achieving 100 percent success in some of my most difficult exams. I could not help but single him out from among my other students. I would, perhaps as unfairly, spend extra time with him, observing and criticizing his laboratory experiments and conclusions. I often remarked, "Bob, you make even my good students look bad."

Needless to say, then, I was bewildered when on the final exam he turned in a completely blank paper. I could only surmise that this was some kind of sad practical joke—certainly strange behavior for such a serious student.

"Bob, this isn't funny," I said. "You know that the final examination counts for two-thirds of your grade."

He just stared at me blankly for a moment and then

walked out of the room. I was both annoyed and baffled, but he never returned with an explanation.

Because of his previous excellence in the subject, I decided, after several debates with my conscience, to give him an "incomplete" in the course instead of the warranted failing grade. I did not see him again for some time, even after the new term commenced. He had apparently dropped out of school.

One day, some weeks later, I met a girlfriend of his in the hallway. She too had been in my chemistry class and greeted me in her usual cheerful manner. I asked if she had seen Bob.

"No, I haven't, Professor Low," she answered. "Bob's been sick. I haven't seen him since his amnesia."

I could not conceal my astonishment, and so she enlightened me.

"I thought everyone knew about it. At the end of last term he had a temporary memory loss," she continued. "It was really spooky. We haven't dated each other since. I still worry about him, though. I can't help it."

"Do you think he'll return to school? He is so gifted and we had become quite good friends."

"I really can't say, Professor Low. I haven't talked to him for some time. He hasn't called me and I'm too proud, I guess, to call him. I did get in touch with him a couple of times several months ago, but he never had much to say. I just assumed that he wasn't interested in me anymore. Maybe you could try. Here, I'll give you his number." She became excited at this suggestion and scrambled in her purse for a scrap of paper. "If you find out anything, will you let me know?"

I promised that I would.

After arguing with myself over whether or not to get

involved, since it really wasn't any of my business, my natural curiosity finally won out, and I called one evening.

"Hello, this is Professor Low from the university. May I speak with Robert Sherman, please?"

"Professor Low, this is Robert." An uncomfortable silence followed. He hadn't sounded very pleased with my call. Finally, I spoke.

"Bob, I've been concerned about you. How are you doing? I hear that you're not well."

He hesitated briefly before beginning his story.

"Professor Low, I've had quite a few health problems lately. I have seen six doctors in four months, and not one of them agrees with the others in the diagnosis. I wish you could see my medicine cabinet." He chuckled. "I could open my own pharmacy. To make matters worse, I get migraine headaches as well. These are even getting worse lately. The truth is, Professor Low, I'm really depressed about the whole thing."

"I can certainly sympathize with you, Bob. Look, I have an idea. I don't know for sure if there's any relationship between your migraines and your other problems, but I'm willing to bet that there is. I can't tell for certain, of course, until we can meet and talk further. Can you see me at the lab tomorrow at about one?"

"Professor Low, I've been through all of this so many times already."

"Bob, please trust me. I've already relieved myself and many others of migraine. Why not give me a chance?"

"Well, I guess it's worth a try. Okay, I'll be there at one."

The following day's meeting proved, to me at least, that my suspicions were correct. Robert had always suffered from migraine, along with its accompanying hypoglycemic symptoms of hunger, weakness, depression, and an insatiable craving for sweets. During the chemistry final he had experienced what his doctors described as "temporary amnesia," brought on by his nervous concern to do well. This was sheer nonsense as far as I was concerned. He had always been overly confident in his knowledge of chemistry. Furthermore, I had never spotted the jitters in him as I had in so many of my other students just before an exam.

"Are you aware that migraine often produces lapses in memory and disorientation?" I asked.

He gestured that he was not.

"Bob, have you ever had a glucose tolerance test done to measure your blood sugar?"

"I'm not positive, but I probably have, judging from the amount of blood that has been taken out of me. I've had them all, from A to Z."

"Would you mind," I asked, "if my laboratory assistant repeated the test? We are equipped to do it right here. We actually do several a week in our research, and the conclusions we've reached have been very interesting."

He shrugged and said that one more test wouldn't matter. I explained that we would take blood samples every fifteen minutes at the beginning of the test, instead of the usual hourly ones, so it might cause him some discomfort. He agreed anyway, and so we scheduled the test for the following morning. I cautioned that he must not eat anything after his meal that evening.

Robert arrived at the prescribed time and, after a sample of blood was taken to determine his fasting blood sugar, he was given a solution of 100 grams of glucose, flavored with lemon to disguise some of the unpleasant taste of so high a concentration of sugar. My assistant then proceeded to take intravenous samples of blood every fifteen minutes and, after a preparatory workup, determined the amount of glucose present in each specimen. After the first hour and a half, we limited our sampling to hourly intervals. Robert's arms had become quite irritated from such frequent venipunctures.

After gathering all the data, I asked my assistant to prepare a graph showing the results. "Bob," I said, "you have the typical curve of a migraine sufferer. It is called the 'flat' glucose tolerance curve and is often mistakenly classified as normal. The shape of this curve is flat only if samples are taken at half- or one-hour intervals—as they usually are [see Figure 6]. Notice that in this 'flat' curve we do not see the initial rise in blood sugar due to the ingestion of the concentrated sugar solution, nor its subsequent drop below normal. However, if we take blood samples at shorter intervals, as we did in your case, we can see the initial rise in the sugar level [see Figure 7]. Let me explain to you what happens in your body to produce this type of glucose tolerance curve."

I then told Robert that in response to the ingestion of sugar, he produces an extraordinarily large amount of insulin very rapidly, much more rapidly than does a hypoglycemic who does not complain of migraine.* This extreme concentration of insulin reduces the level of glucose in the blood almost immediately. It all happens so quickly in most migraine victims that if we wait for one hour before sampling, we completely miss the initial rise in the blood sugar due to the ingestion of the solution of glucose. The high concentration of insulin then stimulates the adrenals to release adrenaline and the other catecholamines just as quickly

---

*The overproduction of insulin by the pancreas of migraine sufferers has actually been measured by the author and found to be much higher than in normal individuals (see pages 112–119 and Figures 12–14). A migraine sufferer can thus have an insulin test directly performed instead of a glucose tolerance test, but its cost is much higher.

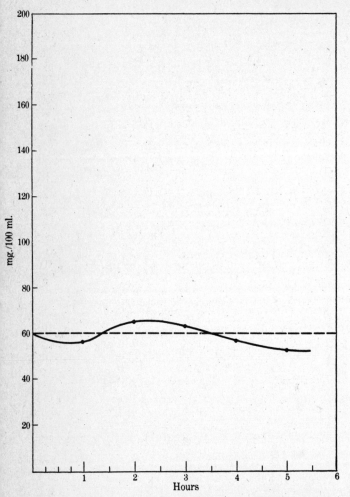

Figure 6. "Flat" curve of a migraine sufferer when blood samples are taken hourly. The initial rise in blood sugar is missed.

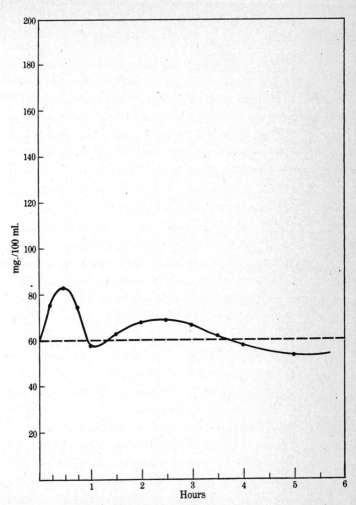

Figure 7. "Flat" curve of a migraine sufferer when blood samples are taken every fifteen minutes for the first hour.

and in similarly high concentrations, destroying most of the insulin and leaving only the necessary amount to reduce the blood sugar level to just slightly below its normal value. This, then, is why the curve is almost flat. The majority of migraine sufferers produce this kind of curve when given a glucose tolerance test.

I explained to Robert how this adrenaline reduces the caliber of the cranial arteries, initiating the migraine attack; how this phenomenon is followed by an expansion of the blood vessels as a consequence of the production by the body of vasodilating prostaglandins, and that this expansion coincides with the initiation of the actual pain.

"Let me see," I continued. "Oh, yes, here's what I'm looking for. This diagram [see Figure 8] illustrates exactly what I just explained to you."

"Professor Low," Robert replied, "this diagram is similar to another one I was looking at while I was getting my tolerance curve done this morning, but it's not exactly the same. Could you clarify the difference for me?"

"Of course. The diagram I'm showing you now illustrates how the adrenals respond to an extraordinarily large amount of insulin. The other diagram [see Figure 5] illustrates how the adrenals respond to low blood sugar. In both cases adrenaline and the other catecholamines are produced and initiate the migraine attack, which in the second case is usually a very severe one. If you eat sugar, your pancreas will produce a large amount of insulin. This diagram [Figure 8] illustrates how the insulin triggers a migraine attack. What you need to do is avoid sugar in your diet.

"Your pancreas is so overactive, however, that even if you don't eat sugar, enough insulin is produced to reduce your blood sugar level below normal after some time, probably after two and a half to three hours. The diagram you saw earlier [Figure 5] illustrates how this triggers a mi-

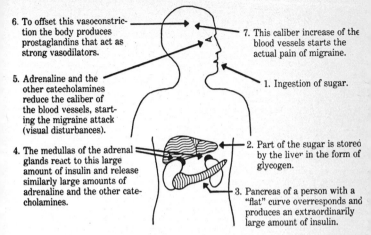

6. To offset this vasoconstriction the body produces prostaglandins that act as strong vasodilators.

7. This caliber increase of the blood vessels starts the actual pain of migraine.

5. Adrenaline and the other catecholamines reduce the caliber of the blood vessels, starting the migraine attack (visual disturbances).

1. Ingestion of sugar.

4. The medullas of the adrenal glands react to this large amount of insulin and release similarly large amounts of adrenaline and the other catecholamines.

2. Part of the sugar is stored by the liver in the form of glycogen.

3. Pancreas of a person with a "flat" curve overresponds and produces an extraordinarily large amount of insulin.

Figure 8. Diagram showing how migraine is produced in an individual suffering from strong hyperinsulinism.

graine attack. You will need to eat at intervals not exceeding two to three hours, and at least six times a day rather than the customary three meals."

"This is fascinating, Professor Low. This morning I read in the notes your assistant showed me while I was waiting that you have triggered migraine attacks by injecting several volunteer students and yourself with one milligram of adrenaline." He kept silent for a few seconds and then his unusual brightness showed up. "Professor Low," he continued, "if the theory you just explained to me is true, then you could as well trigger a migraine attack by injecting insulin, because the body would produce adrenaline by itself."

"Yes, definitely. As far back as 1956, two Italian researchers, Arcangeli and Furian, were able to trigger migraine attacks in each of thirty-one persons suffering from this disease by injecting them with fifteen units of insulin. In contrast to this, twenty-five units of insulin injected into thirty healthy individuals did not initiate an attack in any of them. This certainly suggests that a person must have a predisposition for the disorder for him to fall victim to its distressing symptoms. As you know, the injected insulin starts the counterregulatory mechanism of the body, which causes antagonistic hormones, especially adrenaline, to be secreted. Since adrenaline is ultimately responsible for the triggering of a migraine attack, if this hormone is injected directly into the body of a patient, the symptoms of the disease can also be artificially produced."

Naturally by this time, due to the intake of pure glucose, Bob had the beginnings of a headache. I sent him home with a prescription diet that included six meals a day rich in natural carbohydrates and no refined sugar.

Bob returned to school the following term. His powers of concentration were excellent and he went on after graduation to prove himself in the field of chemistry. Today he is completely free from his attacks of migraine. A few years after he had received his master's degree, I attended the wedding of Robert to Janie Miller, the concerned friend who helped to facilitate his recovery.

Bob's story brings to mind another interesting case. The quality of life of this patient was seriously threatened by a disorder that he did not understand and for which there appeared to be no cure. John Martin, forty-eight years old, had felt constantly tired and nervous since early childhood. When he was sixteen years of age, his migraines began and grew in number and intensity as he got older.

Since his family was poor, he had only a few years of elementary school before he was forced to begin work in a factory. At work he was noted for his punctuality and sense of responsibility, and despite his lack of formal education, his initiative and clever innovations contributed to the quality of the articles he manufactured. Nevertheless, promotion was not to be his reward for quite some time. For no apparent reason, he became negligent to such a degree that he caused damage to the equipment and machinery under his care. His explanation for his mistakes was that he had not been feeling well when they happened; however, the company physician found him to be in perfect health.

As the years passed, his nervousness, fatigue, and headaches increased and he became even more incompetent on the job. One day he had a serious accident, caused by his own carelessness, which led to the amputation of his left arm. Since he was no longer able to perform manual labor, his superiors compassionately made him a foreman in one of the plants. After all, they did feel that he was of above-average intelligence, and they hoped that the new arrangement would benefit both him and the company. But this solution did not work out as they had planned. The man's migraines had become intolerable, and his efficiency diminished significantly.

He was examined by several doctors who could find nothing wrong with him. One of the physicians felt that his troubles stemmed from the loss of his arm and advised him to consult a psychiatrist. Because of the expense involved in this course of treatment, he refused.

When I met him he was in a very bad state, both physically and mentally. A test performed on him proved that he suffered from severe hyperinsulinism. When he was interviewed, it turned out that his diet was very rich in sugars. Breakfast consisted of a heavily sweetened cup of coffee and a slice of bread with jam. His noon and evening meals rarely included a sufficient amount of protein and natural carbohydrates, and he always finished up with a dessert. During the day he snacked on soft drinks, cookies, and cakes.

When his diet was replaced by one high in natural carbohydrates and free from refined sugar, distributed into six meals a day, his improvement was rapid and complete. During the years that I continued to observe him, he did not have a single attack of migraine, his nervousness and fatigue disappeared, and his efficiency on the job increased to such an extent that his superiors promoted him to supervisor. He now earns an excellent salary and is taking night courses at a technical-vocational high school.

7

Refined Versus Natural Sugars

Many years of my life have been dedicated to proving the theory that sugar is indeed the main culprit where migraine is concerned. During this time I have worked closely with many individuals suffering from this disease. Some, of course, were volunteers that I recruited from the student population of the university. Others, however, sought me out after hearing of my successful treatment of migraine. All of them became what one might call my "patients," although I am not a medical doctor. Of these patients, over 90 percent of those who followed my recommendations obtained complete and permanent relief.

I recall that one of my migraine patients, David Barnett, had been instructed by me to eat every two to three hours rather than the customary three meals. In addition, he was to abstain completely from refined sugar and was put on a diet rich in natural carbohydrates, among which were potatoes, rice, breads, crackers, fresh fruits, and unsweetened fruit juices, and also included a sufficient amount of protein. After David had adhered to his "prescription" for three weeks and had experienced total recovery, he came to me bursting with questions.

"Professor Low," he said, "there is something that I don't quite understand about my diet. It works, I know that. But I'm permitted fruit, right?"

"That's correct, David," I replied.

"I've also been drinking fruit juices with my meals and for snacks."

"Unsweetened fruit juices," I corrected.

"That's just my point. Fruit already has sugar in it, right off the tree. If sugar is the major cause of my migraines, why haven't I had one in three weeks?"

"David, when I talk about sugar, I'm referring to it in its refined state; in other words, pure sucrose."

"What's the difference?"

"Well, since you've been relieved of your migraines, apparently there is a big difference. Wouldn't you agree? Your physical and mental health have improved greatly since you began your diet, and yet you are still eating carbohydrates. These are necessary to ensure that your body gets enough glucose for it to function, and to prevent your pancreas from becoming sluggish and eventually atrophic."

"Yes, I understand all of this, but you still haven't answered my question. I have been eating some sugar, as you've just explained, so please enlighten me. Why have my headaches disappeared completely?"

"David, my experiments have shown, time after time, that natural sugars and starch stimulate the pancreas to secrete insulin to a far lesser degree than do their pure counterparts. These results force me to accept the fact that sugars in their natural makeup contain substances that offset their harmful effects on the pancreas. When sugar is refined, these beneficial constituents, supplied by nature's wisdom, are eliminated or destroyed. Here, look at this chart [see Figure 9]. These curves are the average obtained from the tolerance tests of twenty hypoglycemic individuals. You can see that the initial rise in the blood sugar and its subsequent drop are considerably less when natural products are eaten.

"The juices used in this particular study were orange juice and sugarcane juice. I have, however, used other natural fruit juices and obtained identical results. It is also interesting that none of the fruit juices, including the sugarcane juice, produced the symptoms in the hypoglycemic individuals that pure sugar does. Neither did the same unsweetened juices initiate a migraine headache in persons for whom even a very small amount of refined sugar brought on an attack."

"This is all very interesting, Professor Low. What are these substances in natural products that help the hypoglycemic to tolerate sugar?"

"David, I'm sorry to say that I just haven't had time in my research to isolate them. I can only prove this theory by the consistency of my test results. Whatever pure sugar I give to my hypoglycemic volunteers, be it glucose, fructose, sucrose, or maltose, I invariably obtain the same results on a tolerance test. These are always similar to the solid line in the figure that I've just shown you. When natural sugars are given, the results approximate the levels represented by the broken line. My experiments have also shown that the flat curve, typical of an individual suffering from migraine, is much less horizontal after the patient ingests natural sugar than when he eats it in its refined state. This most definitely suggests that natural sugars, unlike purified ones, do not stimulate the pancreas of these individuals to rapidly secrete excessive quantities of insulin.

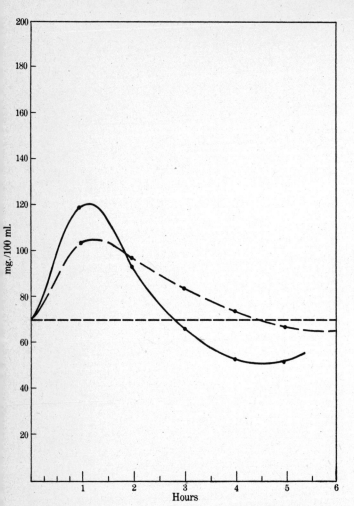

Figure 9. The solid line represents the average blood sugar levels after twenty hypoglycemics ingested 100 grams of glucose. The broken line represents the average blood sugar levels after the same twenty individuals ingested a quantity of fruit juice equivalent to 100 grams of sugar.

It is obvious that in the refining process certain valuable substances are removed from the sugarcane or from the sugar beet. Considering the complexity of the technology involved in sugar refining, one can easily see how many of nature's ingredients can be lost. Since pure, refined sugar is devoid of all vitamins, minerals, and proteins, some of these are doubtless the constituents that must be preserved if sugar is to be metabolized properly. An apple, although it is rich in its own sugar, also contains many vitamins and other nutrients. A migraine sufferer, therefore, can eat it and experience no discomfort. It raises many interesting questions, wouldn't you say? David, if anyone could isolate these components, the migraine patient probably wouldn't be forced to eliminate sweets from his diet. However, until this becomes a reality, he has no other choice if he wishes to maintain his health."

"Professor Low, this reminds me of how certain diseases can be caused by vitamin deficiencies. I'm thinking of how scurvy was once a widespread and dangerous illness, feared by sailors as much as a stormy sea. And just think how easy it was to cure the disease once man stumbled onto the answer."

"Yes, David, it wasn't until oranges and limes were introduced to the ship's galley that the problem was solved, although no one knew of vitamin C at that time. Nutrition is a very exciting field to pursue in the treatment and prevention of disease. Do you recall the story of vitamin B?" I went on to relate one of my favorite tales.

"Toward the end of the last century, beriberi was ravaging the hospitals and jails of the Dutch East Indies. It was initially believed that a microbe was the causative agent, but none could ever be isolated. Quite by accident, it was discovered that persons eating polished white rice contracted the disease, but that the natives, who ate the rough brown paddy rice, did not. It was thought then that the rice chaff contained an antidote for the disease. It was only later, about 1911, that Casimir Funk isolated vitamin B_1 from the rice chaff. This led to the conclusion that a deficiency in this vitamin was the cause of beriberi.

"Other researchers came to a similar conclusion when they discovered that a food prepared with the optimal amounts of purified proteins, fats, carbohydrates, and minerals required by the body caused the disease known as 'night blindness,' whereas the ailment did not occur if the same ingredients were used in an unpurified form. Once the findings of Casimir Funk were known, it was also possible to establish that the illness was caused by the lack of a substance necessary to the proper functioning of the body, vitamin A. Soon it was found that other illnesses such as scurvy, pellagra, and rickets occurred because components essential to health—the vitamins—had been removed from various foods consumed in modern societies.

"Not long ago I read a book by Herbert Bailey that describes a number of experiments conducted by two Canadians, Evan Shute and Wilfred Shute. Their work parallels what we have been discussing. They propose that a lack of vitamin E in our modern diet is responsible in part for the high incidence of heart disease that we have today. Unlike our ancestors, most of us in the twentieth century prefer white flour rather than whole wheat for baking. In the preparation of this more refined white flour, the wheat germ and many of the vitamins that enrich it are removed. To make matters worse, the final product is then bleached for aesthetic purposes. Wheat germ is an important source of vitamin E, and since this is eliminated from the flour in order to lengthen the shelf life of the products made with it, many individuals may not be getting all of the vitamin E required by their bodies.

"According to Evan and Wilfred Shute, vitamin E, or alphatocopherol, is a natural oxygen conservator that has many beneficial effects on the body. When provided with vitamin E, healthy cells do not need as much oxygen and so the excess is directed to those parts of the body that are in greater need of it. A diseased heart, after receiving enough vitamin E, can rest and restore itself since it doesn't have to pump as hard to transport blood to the cells of the body. Also, the ailing heart itself is more adequately supplied with the oxygen needed for its repair.

"Vitamin E appears to have other properties as well that can greatly help an individual suffering from cardiovascular disease. The vitamin apparently acts as a vasodilator, opening the arteries so that the blood flows more easily. In a disease such as atherosclerosis, this can be very significant. According to the advocates of vitamin E, it also acts as an anticoagulant and thus helps to prevent clots.

"The Shutes claim remarkable results in their treatment of heart disease by employing vitamin E therapy. Scarring is a major problem following a heart attack, sometimes rendering a region of the heart useless because of the reduced blood supply to a section of the muscle. Treatment with vitamin E during the healing process has apparently prevented this formation of scar tissue. A word of caution, however: an excess of vitamin E, as any excess, can be harmful to the patient.

"Disease need not be cured by drugs alone, after all. More and more research money is being channeled into studies of what we eat or do not eat as possible causes of disease. Certain food additives have already been taken off the market due to their carcinogenic properties. Before we get too far off the subject, there is something else that I'd like you to see." I found the chart that I wanted and showed it to David (see Figure 10).

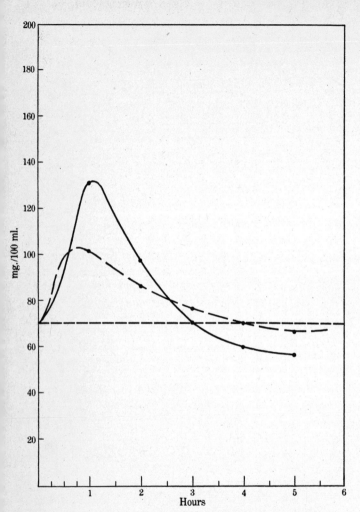

Figure 10. *The solid line represents the average blood sugar levels after twenty hypoglycemics ingested 100 grams of pure starch. The broken line represents the average blood sugar levels after the same twenty individuals ingested an amount of whole wheat bread equivalent to 100 grams of starch.*

"Once again we have the averages of the tolerance tests of twenty hypoglycemic patients. The solid line represents the blood sugar levels after the ingestion of one hundred grams of pure starch. The broken line pictures the levels after the ingestion of an equivalent amount of starch contained in whole wheat bread. Can you see the incredible difference in the way in which the two influence the blood sugar? The whole wheat bread is a far weaker pancreatic stimulator than is the pure starch. Between these two extremes, of the pure starch, which is never found outside a chemical lab, and the whole wheat, a highly beneficial food substance, there is white flour. Although it has been stripped of many of its natural ingredients, some do remain, so that the migraine patient is able to tolerate this carbohydrate. He can likewise eat spaghetti and polished white rice without being subject to migraine attack. This leads to the conclusion that some of the natural constituents necessary for proper metabolism by the hypoglycemic do remain after the flour is processed. Of course, the ideal would definitely be the whole wheat flour, but white flour does not bring on a migraine.

"Wouldn't it be a great contribution to mankind if someone could find a way of processing sugar so that all of nature's elements would be preserved? Rather than worry about its whiteness and purity, manufacturers would do better to concern themselves with the retention of all of sugar's natural components. This would, of course, involve changing over from the present technology to a new and better method. Perhaps lyophilization, or freeze-drying, of the sugarcane juice would be the answer. This is a drying process in which water contained in a product is first frozen and then vaporized, without passing through the liquid state. Freeze-dried products completely recover their original properties when water is added to them. The public itself must begin to insist on a better quality of food, a more natural food, and worry less about aesthetics and convenience. After all, our good health is the most important gift that we have, and we should do everything in our power to preserve it."

My conversation with David brought to mind a man I had treated who unfortunately had carried my advice to the extreme. When I met him, he was forty-three years old and had suffered the pain of migraine since he was fifteen. When he was just a sophomore in college, his father, the owner of a very successful commercial firm, died of a heart attack. Since my patient was the oldest son in the family, he had to give up his studies in order to take charge of the business and provide a means of support for the rest of the family. At first he was quite competent at his new job, but little by little, problems began to arise that he was not capable of solving, and in just a few years the family firm went bankrupt.

This man was always irritable, tired, and depressed, and his indulgence in sweets could not be controlled. His migraines, which had begun early in his life, occurred with increasing frequency, sometimes as often as twice a week. He seemed destined to suffer one calamity after another: after the bankruptcy of the family business, his irascible behavior and heavy drinking led his wife, to whom he had been married only a few years, to abandon him. His health worsened at an alarming rate, probably due to his excessive indulgence in sweets, alcohol, and cigarettes. He was an individual with no moderation; everything he did was marked by extremes.

Finally, after losing his fourth job in one year, he sought medical help. The test administered to him showed that he suffered from strong hyperinsulinism. Since the man's doctor happened to be a good friend of mine and was well aware of my successful work with migraine patients, he referred his patient to me for diet therapy. I provided him with my usual advice—frequent meals high in natural carbohydrates and devoid of sugar—and also suggested that he give up the alcohol of which he had become so fond. The man seemed very earnest in his attempt to reform his life. He assured me that he would do everything that was necessary to live once again like a normal person.

I was very surprised then when, after six months had passed, I received a call from the man's doctor. He told me that his patient had been cured of his migraines but was now suffering from a vitamin deficiency. It seems that the patient, as he had done with everything else in his life, had carried my advice about avoiding sugar to an unhealthy extreme. He had apparently tuned out my lecture on the difference between refined and natural carbohydrates. He had given up not only refined sugar but also fresh fruits and juices as well, and since he had never cared for vegetables, his body was in dire need of the vitamins that these natural carbohydrates can provide. His mistake was that he lumped all carbohydrates together. When he began to follow my diet as it had been written, his health was completely restored. Today he occupies an important position as director of a well-known firm.

8

Migraine and Drugs

It should be clear by now that no medicines are necessary to prevent migraine attacks. This can be accomplished by avoiding the ingestion of processed sugars and following the other recommendations given in this book.

It is, however, interesting for the reader to know the effect that drugs can have on migraine sufferers because, as explained below, many medicines may even worsen their condition.

Medical history teaches that man from time immemorial has tried to cure his diseases by the ingestion of all kinds of extraneous substances. Ancient medical writings tell of exotic formulas that have their counterpart in modern synthetic chemical products—vaccines, serums, hormones, vitamins, and antibiotics—but the tendency to treat ailments by the introduction into the body of substances that are foreign to it remains the same today as it was in the past. Without ignoring the tremendous benefits of these medications to mankind, it should not be forgotten that, in addition to their therapeutic action, they can also have side effects harmful to the human organism. In the treatment of illnesses, it is therefore necessary to be ever alert, so that these medicines can be discontinued or changed if the side effects appear to constitute any danger.

Until Louis Pasteur's discovery, in the last half of the nineteenth century, that microbes cause many of the prevalent diseases, it was generally thought that poisons caused all ailments, and drugs were widely used as antidotes. When, at the beginning of this century, Paul Ehrlich discovered that the drug salvarsan was a cure for syphilis, the idea of treating illnesses by introducing foreign substances into the body gained further support.

A new era in medicine began when it was discovered that afflictions such as beriberi, scurvy, rickets, night blindness, and pellagra were caused not by poisons or microbes but by the lack of certain substances essential to the functioning of the human body—vitamins. This change in firmly established patterns of thinking was difficult for many to accept, but the evidence that these ailments were indeed curable through the use of vitamins B, C, D, and A and nicotinic acid, respectively, was irrefutable. Although vitamins are not "foreign" to the human body, the newly discovered illnesses were cured by introducing them into the body.

In light of this long tradition of curing illnesses by administering medications, it was only logical that drugs have been used to try to cure migraine headache. But at this point medical science admits that the cause of this disease is unknown. Therefore all efforts to find a medication to cure it have been unsuccessful. The purpose of medicines in common current use for migraine is to lessen the severity of the attacks; they are mainly painkillers, vasoconstrictors, or antiserotonin substances. The most commonly used painkiller is aspirin, which, as we shall see, may in some instances worsen the pain.

Ergotamine tartrate is widely used as a vasoconstrictor and, if taken in the prepain stage, can sometimes abort the headache or at least reduce the pain. In most cases, however, it has no effect at all. Ergotamine tartrate is contraindicated in hypertension, cardiovascular disease, thrombophlebitis, and renal disease.

Methysergide, an antiserotonin drug, has prevented attacks in some cases, at the risk, however, of causing extremely serious side effects, such as retroperitoneal fibrosis and urethral obstruction. In addition, it has the same contraindications as ergotamine tartrate.

Another drug, now widely used to control migraine, is propranolol (Inderal). A number of migraine sufferers claim that they have noticed some relief by its use, but for many of them the side effects are very disagreeable. Other drugs, under testing at this time, do not give much hope either.

Drugs That Curb the Activity of the Pancreas

As migraine headache is a consequence of hyperinsulinism, or an overactive pancreas, any drug able to curb the activity of this organ should also be able to prevent migraine attacks.

Many drugs have been tested to control the insulin secretion by the pancreas, but the effect of most of them has proved to be either dangerous or ineffective. High hopes are now being placed on a recently discovered drug, known as diazoxide, or chloromethylbenzothiadiazine. However, the use of this drug is still in the experimental stage, and it appears to result in side effects that have not yet been brought under control.

Drugs That Can Stimulate the Pancreas to Secrete Insulin

Aspirin, or acetylsalicylic acid, is the leading over-the-counter painkiller. This drug and other painkillers alleviate headaches by inhibiting the synthesis of vasodilating prostaglandins. If aspirin is used in large doses, however, it may extend the duration of a migraine attack or contribute to the initiation of another one because it can in itself cause the pancreas to release insulin—just what the migraine patient doesn't need! Although it is not well known for this action, a large dose of aspirin actually multiplies the detrimental effect of sugar by further increasing the output of insulin.

A young woman I met recently told me of her uncle's long-time struggle with migraine. For as long as she could remember, and certainly since she was a young child (at the time of our meeting she was thirty-three), she recalled that he would spend two or three days in bed with the illness. Her aunt would always caution her to be very quiet, because "Uncle Carl has one of his headaches." All brands of painkillers containing aspirin were constantly on hand and the man carried a bottle with him wherever he went, "just in case." Yet he seemed always to be laid up with the excruciating pain of his migraines. Sometimes, much to the horror of her aunt, who was herself suspicious of all drugs, he would pop as many as four or five tablets at a time. However, not even this many pills gave him any satisfactory relief. As I explained to the young woman, since aspirin is one of the salicylates, it was actually complicating his already serious hypoglycemic condition.

In fact, the knowledge that some medications have a stimulating effect on the pancreas has become a very important factor in the effort to relieve migraine. Synthetic drugs known as hypoglycemic drugs have been developed to be used in lieu of insulin in the treatment of diabetes; the most important of these are the sulfonylurea derivatives, such as tolbutamide. These medicines incite the pancreas to increase its insulin output. Many other synthetic drugs, used in the treatment of different diseases, also have hypoglycemic effects. Obviously if persons suffering from hyperinsulinism take one of these drugs, their condition would grow worse. To avoid any risk they should abstain from any drug that is not indispensable for the control of other ailments; and constant care must be exercised to observe any side effects of drugs it is impossible to omit. In the event of a hypoglycemic reaction, or if such an effect is even suspected, the patient should contact his doctor, who will decide if the drug must be discontinued or if it can be replaced by another one of comparable therapeutic action but without this side effect.

During our talk, the young woman enthusiastically took notes on all aspects of the proper diet, and I prepared a list for her of all known drugs and chemicals that can initiate an attack of migraine. I received a letter from her two months later and I was happy to learn that her uncle was enjoying the best of health.

The hypoglycemic effect of medications is especially evident when two of them are administered simultaneously, since their effects are mutually reinforced. This is the case with a well-known prescription painkiller, widely used to alleviate the pain of many discomforts and sometimes also used by migraine patients. It is composed of two drugs, propoxyphene and aspirin, both of which, while actually able to ease pain, also stimulate the pancreas to secrete insulin. Unlike aspirin, however, this drug can be purchased only with a doctor's prescription and so there is less danger to the migraine sufferer from its misuse than from aspirin.

It is wise, nevertheless, to be aware that this medicine, while giving temporary relief to the pain of migraine, can increase the frequency and intensity of the attacks.

The following case is an example of drug-induced hypoglycemia from yet another medication.

Helen Mitchell, age forty-seven, had her first attack of migraine when she was only thirteen years old. Her family history showed that her father and one of her brothers had also complained of the disorder—which raises another interesting aspect of migraine, that of heredity, that will be discussed later on in the book. Once I had placed Helen on a strict diet of frequent, sugar-free meals, I anticipated that her problems would disappear in a short time, as had happened in all other cases I dealt with. I was quite surprised, therefore, when she experienced only partial improvement. I then began an investigation to identify any possible hypoglycemic element that might have been overlooked in her diet; but, despite intense questioning, Helen still was unable to enlighten me. She promised that she had faithfully adhered to the necessary eating habits and had taken no medications for migraine. She became an intriguing mystery to my staff and myself. Finally, after yet another thorough interrogation, she admitted that she sometimes took one of the popular sleeping pills. Apparently she had felt that this was too insignificant to mention, since the drug was not taken on a regular basis. I had previously researched the hypnotic that Helen was taking, a nitrobenzodiazepine derivative, and found it to be hypogylcemic in nature. When Helen gave up the suspected drug, she experienced immediate and total relief from the discomfort of migraine.

I can also recall the case of Harry Blake, a student at the university where I had taught for so many years and also held the position of dean. I had not been associated with the university for some time when I met Harry, but a professor with whom I had kept in touch recommended that he come to see me. My old friend, the professor, knew that I was completely involved in migraine research by this time and felt that I might help this young student. Harry Blake had been a victim of migraine for seven years and had undergone the usual number of medical tests without success, as well as several expensive and fruitless sessions with a psychiatrist. After reviewing his case history, I elected not to perform the diagnostic glucose tolerance test, although I was sure he had not undergone one previously. Since his symptoms indicated that he was a classic case of hyperinsulinism complicated by migraine, I was convinced that if I had tested him he would produce the typical flat curve. I decided, therefore, to eliminate what I considered the needless discomfort of the test and go straight to the diet therapy. If my suspicions that he suffered from low blood sugar were correct, the specialized diet would rid him of his symptoms and thus prove the accuracy of my diagnosis.

I recommended the usual dietary regimen and sent him on his way, convinced that he soon would join the ranks of those who had been relieved. After two months had passed, he unexpectedly returned to me with the same complaints. Harry explained that after being on his diet for several weeks he had felt better than he had in years. Lately, however, for some unknown reason his migraines had returned. We sat down together for an in-depth discussion and finally uncovered his problem. Harry had developed a bacterial infection, for which he had been taking an antibiotic, oxytetracycline, for about two weeks prior to our second meeting. I explained to Harry that this was indeed the root of his recent troubles, since oxytetracycline has hypoglycemic properties and so is capable of stimulating the pancreas to secrete insulin. Since the infection had cleared up nicely,

Harry's doctor took him off the prescription. He recovered completely after that, according to my friend, his teacher.

If a migraine patient finds that the prescribed treatment has not provided total relief, he should begin to question any medication that he may be taking at the time. Furthermore, if a relapse in his condition closely coincides with a specific medical treatment, he should discuss this condition with his doctor. Most physicians should be willing to prescribe a substitute medication (which in most cases is readily available) that has equivalent therapeutic value but no hypoglycemic effects. Since the average patient does not know the chemicals included in a specific medication, the following tables of hypoglycemic drugs—drugs that can increase the output of insulin by the pancreas—may help him to address the necessary questions to his physician. Table 2 (on page 84) lists hypoglycemic drugs that have been previously cited for that effect in medical literature. Table 3 (on page 85) includes hypoglycemic drugs that I have not found credited as such in the literature but that I myself have observed to have hypoglycemic effects.

Other Substances That Adversely Affect the Migraine Sufferer

Alcohol

Recent studies have shown that alcohol has a strong hypoglycemic effect; this is because it interferes with the function of the liver, which regulates carbohydrate metabolism. Many healthy persons can easily tolerate reasonable amounts of alcohol, but unfortunately the same cannot be said for the victims of hypoglycemia. Such persons must therefore abstain from alcoholic beverages, especially the most concentrated ones such as bourbon, brandy, cognac, gin, rye,

Table 2. Drugs with hypoglycemic effect that have been mentioned in medical literature

Chemical name	Use	Observations
bishydroxycoumarin	anticoagulant	moderately hypoglycemic if used alone, but strongly hypoglycemic if used with sulfonylureas
chlorpromazine	in psychiatric practice, especially against excitement	
oxytetracycline	broad-spectrum antibiotic	
phenylbutazone	anti-inflammatory drug, mainly used against rheumatic fever and rheumatoid arthritis	moderately hypoglycemic if used alone, but strongly hypoglycemic if used with sulfonylureas
propoxyphene	painkiller	Darvon is a mixture of propoxyphene and aspirin.
salicylates	painkiller and anti-inflammatory; widely used against rheumatic fever and rheumatoid arthritis	Aspirin is acetylsalicylic acid.
sulfisoxazole	antimicrobial	moderately hypoglycemic if used alone, but strongly hypoglycemic if used with sulfonylureas
sulfonylureas	to treat diabetes	The most widely used are: Acetohexamide, Chlorpropamide, Tolazamide, and tolbutamide.
phenformin	to treat diabetes	

Table 3. Drugs that have been proved by the author to be hypoglycemic in nature

Chemical name	Use	Observations
nitrobenzodiazepine derivative	to treat insomnia	
oxyquinazoline	to treat insomnia	
calcium gluconate	against osteoporosis and whenever increased calcium intake is required	The pancreatic stimulator is the gluconate ion, not the calcium ion.
corticosteroids	anti-inflammatory drugs, mainly used against rheumatic fever and rheumatoid arthritis	
isobuthyl-phenylpropionic acid (Ibuprofen)	anti-inflammatory drug, also used as a painkiller	

NOTE: Many other drugs are being investigated for their hypoglycemic nature.

scotch, vodka, and whiskey. Sweet wines and liqueurs are highly detrimental to the hypoglycemic and their ingestion almost always precipitates migraine attacks in predisposed persons. This is due to the combined presence in these drinks of two strongly hypoglycemic substances, alcohol and sugar, the effects of which are mutually reinforced. Beer is even more harmful than sweet wines and liqueurs because it contains at least three substances whose hypoglycemic effects mutually reinforce one another: maltose, alcohol, and oxalic acid.

The hard liquors contain no sugar, but their alcoholic content is high, from 34 to 45 percent. Beer and ale contain only about 5 percent alcohol but are loaded with maltose, a highly detrimental carbohydrate for the hypoglycemic. Dry table wines, such as burgundies, clarets and sauternes, usually contain from 8 to 8.5 percent alcohol. Sherry, port, and Madeira contain a much higher percentage, usually between 15 and 20 percent; they also contain a large amount of sugar.

You can see why it is best for a migraine patient to avoid all of these potent drinks with the possible exception of an occasional glass of dry table wine with a meal.

Caffeine

A distant cousin of mine visited me several years ago and stayed with my family for eight weeks. Since we had many years on which to catch up, he and I enjoyed endless discussions that sometimes lasted well into the night. I was interested to discover that he too had been victimized by migraine from an early age. I explained my work to him, and during his stay he agreed to try my treatment. His condition did improve somewhat in the course of his visit, but he still experienced several mild attacks. I was baffled at first, until he admitted that he was in the habit of drinking seven or eight cups of strong coffee each day—something I hadn't noticed since most of my day was spent at the laboratory. When he reduced his coffee consumption to three cups of a weaker brew per day, he was relieved of all of his migraine attacks.

Caffeine does not directly stimulate the pancreas to secrete insulin, but rather acts on the adrenal glands. Thus caffeine skips the first step in the making of a migraine and goes directly to the second—the release of adrenaline and the other catecholamines. You will recall that adrenaline is capable of converting glycogen into glucose and releasing it into the bloodstream. Consequently, if a hypoglycemic individual drinks a beverage containing both sugar and caffeine, like sweetened coffee or one of the many soft drinks containing these two ingredients, the concentration of glucose in his blood will increase for two reasons: (1) because the sugar that is eaten directly is completely converted into glucose, and (2) because the glycogen stored in the liver is transformed into glucose. This double effect brings about a still greater increase in the production of insulin. Like the caffeine, the insulin stimulates the adrenals to release their hormones; and we all know the ending to this story for the migraine sufferer.

9

Mental Disorder and Migraine

One of my most interesting cases was that of Jane Baker, who now heads the department of humanities at a leading university. When we first met, however, she did not hold this prestigious position. She was in fact still in the process of recovering from a nervous breakdown that she had experienced ten years before.

Our meeting was not exactly by chance. At a Christmas social, I met Jane's sister. We chatted about my work, which eventually led to the telling of her sister's long, sad story.

"My sister has migraines quite often," Jane's sister told me, "but hers began as the result of a severe shock that she suffered when she was only twenty-two. She's never completely recovered and that's why her headaches persist. I really can't believe that they're due to low blood sugar because she never had them before her breakdown."

I defended my position, without even knowing all of the facts. "Emotional upsets may cause the pituitary gland to produce certain hormones that in their turn stimulate the pancreas to generate insulin," I argued. "A slightly overactive pancreas can thus become overactive enough to trigger migraine attacks in predisposed individuals."

"Yes, but how do you explain the fact that the migraines never occurred previously?" she asked.

"Well, perhaps to answer the question accurately, I should be told all of the details. What was this great shock that changed your sister's life so drastically?"

It was an unusual tale:

"When my sister was only twenty-two, she became engaged to be married. Peter was a wonderful young man and Jane was very much in love with him. One evening, two weeks before the wedding was to take place, they attended a friend's birthday party, accompanied by another couple. The party was held away from the city in a lonely sector of town. After the festivities, my sister and Peter, along with the other couple, started for home. It was very late, about two in the morning. After about fifteen minutes had passed, Peter informed everyone that he had been watching a car in the rearview mirror that seemed to be following them. Unfortunately, this proved to be correct. Shortly afterward the car passed them and screeched to a stop horizontally in front of them, blocking their way. Four men jumped out and two of them carried guns. Peter immediately jerked the car into reverse and stepped on the gas, turning at the first crossroad. The other car pursued them closely. Peter told the others that he would try to get to town and the nearest police station. When they had just reached the limits of the city, they were horrified when their pursuers began to shoot at them, probably in an attempt to stop their car. They all evaded the bullets by ducking below the seats, but since Peter was driving and could not duck, he was hit in the head. The car skidded, but the other gentleman, acting quickly, took the wheel. They stopped only half a block from the police station, as the other car sped away. Peter was pronounced dead fifteen minutes later in the emergency room of the hospital. Jane hasn't been the same since."

"Is this, then, when the migraines began?"

"Yes. Naturally, she developed many other problems as well."

"Other problems? What exactly do you mean?"

"She had what the doctors diagnosed as a nervous break-down. She couldn't sleep or eat and cried constantly, even months after Peter was buried. She dropped out of school and spent six months in a sanatorium. She improved enough to be released and we insisted that she try to continue with her education; we felt that this would help her to forget the tragedy. She did manage to go as far as her master's, but it took her many years to accomplish this. It wasn't an easy task for her, although she is a very intelligent girl. Jane's studies were interrupted many times due to her unbalanced psychological state and poor physical condition, which plagued her with frequent and intense migraines."

"I'd like to meet Jane," I said. "I can't guarantee any-thing, but I think I can eliminate her headaches and perhaps many of her other difficulties. Your sister's migraines were, in all probability, triggered by the tragedy, but she was always predisposed to them. As I told you before, emotional disorders can indirectly stimulate the pancreas of an indi-vidual to increase its production of insulin. In Jane's case her body overresponds, causing her already overactive pan-creas to generate enough insulin to trigger an attack. Jane's poor diet in the years following her breakdown contributed to her hypoglycemia and her neurotic state."

Jane's sister agreed that it was worth pursuing the pos-sibility that I was right. A week later I was contacted by

Jane. We met on the following day and talked for almost two hours. She explained that she was also troubled with sleepiness, but attributed this to the many tranquilizers that she was taking. Furthermore, her hunger could not be satiated, although she did not gain weight. Jane was seeing a psychiatrist on a regular basis; anxiety and depression seemed always to be a part of her makeup, and her migraines were getting worse, not better.

Later that same week, we performed an insulin test. When Jane had seen the results—her curve was typical of an individual with migraine—she became convinced that my diagnosis was sound.

I explained that she must give up refined sugar and all products made with it and eat every two to three hours. I also told her to ask her doctor to reduce the doses of tranquilizers. She did as I asked, and her improvement was rapid. Her headaches occurred less frequently and, when they did, were less intense. After a month or so, she took herself off the tranquilizers altogether; and after just ten weeks, she was completely relieved of all her physical problems. Her attitude has also improved considerably, and, although she will never be able to forget completely the tragedy that had triggered her breakdown, she is now beginning to live with it behind her. Her mental restoration lends credence to the old proverb "A sound mind in a sound body." In addition to holding an important academic position in one of the leading universities, she has recently become engaged to a young professor of sociology.

There is a growing tendency to attribute "difficult to diagnose" physical disorders to an individual's mental state. Much is heard about psychosomatic illnesses, but very little about "somatopsychic" ones. It is very significant that some of the more common symptoms of hypoglycemia are anxiety, depression, a propensity to cry, fatigue, irritability, insomnia, indecision, thoughts of suicide, temper, fear, and nausea. More often than not, a patient with such problems would automatically be diagnosed as neurotic or even psychotic.

It was generally thought in the past that neuroses and other psychic disorders could easily be differentiated from hypoglycemia because in the former condition the patient is usually free from feelings of constant intense hunger and unusual craving for sweets. But there are studies that suggest that many persons suffering from depression, anxieties, compulsions, phobias, and other mental diseases would prove to be victims of hyperinsulinism, if the appropriate test were performed on them. Furthermore, a hypoglycemic condition that is capable of producing a variety of psychological disorders need not always be accompanied by the classic symptoms of fatigue and insatiable hunger. It has been found that the symptoms of various psychic disorders can be alleviated and the conditions permanently cured in a great number of cases by employing the proper diet.

I remember another woman, Emily Keegan, who had undergone psychiatric counseling for twenty years, since the age of seventeen. For no apparent reason, from time to time a feeling of overwhelming terror would consume her, and would lead to attacks of severe nausea and stomach pains. These spells became more and more frequent as she grew older, and she was forced to give up her job and seek unemployment compensation. Although a battery of tests had been conducted on her over the years to determine a physical cause for her complaints, her condition was invariably diagnosed as psychological in nature. She was so distressed over her health that she even put herself under regressive hypnosis in an attempt to discover the origin of her problems, but nothing was uncovered. Ms. Keegan became inordinately afraid to leave her home for any length of time because of the embarrassment her attacks could cause her. Quite by chance, she found that if she carried snacks with her whenever she went out and ate something every two hours, she could bypass her fear attacks and the other discomforts that she usually suffered. When, finally, an alert and well-informed psychiatrist suggested that she have an insulin or glucose tolerance test performed, it was found that she did indeed suffer from hyperinsulinism. This is now being corrected with the proper diet, and she is beginning to enjoy life once again.

In 1935 G. B. Lake, editor of the journal *Clinical Medicine and Surgery*, wrote:

It now seems highly probable that within the next five or ten years, the physician who attempts to treat any case of psychic disorder, from the mildest neurosis or irregularity of behavior to the severest type of psychosis, without the help of one or several blood studies, will be looked upon as a heedless blunderer who is no credit to his profession.

Today, over fifty years later, this prediction has unfortunately not been fulfilled.

10

Some Interesting Facts About Migraine

A Difficult Case

One of my most curious patients was a man who at age thirty-nine had already achieved his life's goal of becoming president of the company for which he had worked since college. During his first year in this prestigious job the firm enjoyed considerable prosperity, due to the intelligence of his leadership and his competency in decision making. When I met Donald Gibbs, I found him to be in a state of depression, physically exhausted, and suffering from frequent attacks of migraine. During his second year in command, his behavior had quite suddenly begun to change. He vacillated on major policies, leaving the fate of his company to less knowledgeable subordinates. Consequently, the prosperity of the firm decreased substantially. It was this unfortunate turn of events that forced him to seek the advice of his doctor, who prescribed tranquilizers and counseled him to take a long vacation, away from the pressures of his job. Mr. Gibbs followed this advice, but later, when he returned to work after his therapeutic rest, he found that his condition had not improved. Furthermore, his migraines, which had begun two years earlier, grew worse.

Since all his physical examinations and laboratory tests had produced only negative results, his doctor advised him to see a psychoanalyst. This specialist was of the opinion that Mr. Gibbs was seeking an escape from his enormous responsibilities and that this was giving him his headaches. He therefore advised his patient to seek a less demanding position away from his present place of employment. He was taking his first steps in this direction when we happened to meet.

Mr. Gibbs had been invited by the university to be the guest speaker at Business Administration Day. I wasn't directly involved in the occasion, but a fellow teacher asked me to attend. At a luncheon, after the speeches and formalities were over, I met and chatted with the guest of honor. Our conversation wandered to my field of interest, and thus fate led another victim of migraine to me.

A glucose tolerance test showed that his blood sugar level initially rose to a normal height, but after five hours dropped to more than 25 percent below the fasting level. Had the test been limited to three or four hours, this latent hypoglycemia would have been missed. Mr. Gibbs is one of the not-too-frequent migraine victims who do not produce the characteristic flat curve when tested. His case proves the necessity of prolonging the test to five hours for certain individuals in order to pick up their hypoglycemia (see Figure 11).

I showed the results to Mr. Gibbs and made the usual recommendations.

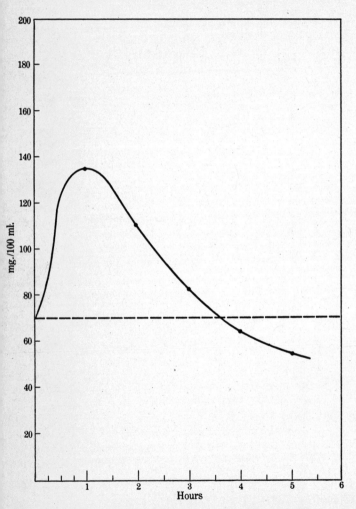

Figure 11. Blood sugar curve of Mr. Donald Gibbs.

"Mr. Gibbs," I said, "it is essential that you eliminate all processed sugars from your diet."

"But Professor Low, I never eat any sugar."

"Surely you must eat some sweets or desserts?"

He shook his head.

"Perhaps you use sugar in your coffee or tea?" I insisted.

"No, I never eat sweets of any kind. You see, I learned to do without sugar when I was just a boy. My teeth are very prone to cavities and so I was not permitted to eat treats made with sugar, and now I find that I've even lost a taste for them. I am proud of the fact that I still have all of my own teeth."

I have to admit that I was baffled. I then remembered that when we had eaten lunch together at the time of our first meeting, his beverage had been beer.

"Mr. Gibbs, I hope you don't mind this question, but I must ask it," I continued. "Do you drink much beer?"

He admitted that for some time he had been enjoying three or four bottles of beer a day, usually with his meals.

"This then is the cause of your troubles," I said.

He was naturally skeptical that his moderate drinking caused any harm, but admitted that the beginning of his attacks of migraine coincided closely with his increased fondness for beer. I advised him to do without this beverage, and when he did this his condition improved in a few weeks.

Mr. Gibbs is once again directing a profitable company with the ability that he had initially shown. His case proves the necessity of eliminating all processed sugars from the diet of a migraine victim. All refined sugars act on the pancreas in the same way, including the maltose found in beer. Furthermore, as explained in Chapter 8, beer also contains alcohol and oxalic acid, and the hypoglycemic effects of these substances are mutually reinforced. Beer is

especially detrimental to the migraine sufferer and therefore must be avoided at all costs.

The Weekend Headache

Migraine has been attributed for years to the tensions and
pressures of everyday life. Isn't it unusual then that in many
people attacks take place mainly on weekends or on holi-
days, that is, precisely when the patients are at rest and
away from the stress of their jobs?

As far back as 1949, C. F. Wilkinson, Jr., in a paper
published in the *American Journal of the Medical Sciences*,
described a patient who had attacks of migraine only on
Sundays. It was discovered that on weekdays the man's
breakfast consisted of bacon and eggs, while on Sundays he
treated himself to waffles and syrup. I have encountered
many similar cases. An example is that of Evelyn Havens,
who worked for a busy advertising agency as an account
executive. She put in long and sometimes tense hours during the week, and yet, while predisposed to migraine, she
never experienced any of its symptoms at work. On weekends, however, more often than not, she suffered from severe headaches. Evelyn was an easygoing person by nature
and so was able to relax on her days off and forget her job.
Naturally, then, she was perplexed by her strange migraine
pattern.

Together we investigated her habits, and eventually a
pattern came to light. During the week her meals were
nutritious but light and always excluded desserts. Her
physical appearance was important to her job and so she
carefully watched her weight. On weekends she "let her
hair down," and splurged with alcoholic drinks, desserts,
and sweet snacks. Evelyn almost always paid the price for
these luxuries with a pounding Sunday headache.

Sometimes migraine attacks occur periodically in a pattern that does not coincide with the weekend. In such cases, it can usually be proved that the diets of the patients involved contain more sugar precisely on the days of the week when the attacks occur.

When Else?

As we have already seen, a migraine sufferer cannot abstain from eating for more than two to three hours without experiencing an attack. His pancreas is usually so overactive that even without the stimulation of sugar or any other hypoglycemic substance, a quantity of insulin is produced after a certain period of time that is sufficient to trigger an attack. Fasting for more than two to three hours must therefore be avoided. For the same reason it is equally important for the migraine patient to eat a snack before going to bed. Otherwise it is possible that he will awake in the morning in severe pain. In extreme cases it is even necessary to set the alarm and awake during the night for a snack. A couple of crackers would suffice.

Unlike the hypoglycemic, a healthy person can pass a substantial period of time without eating before the level of glucose in his blood drops below normal. Furthermore, the hunger he experiences, even after several days of fasting, is significantly less than that felt by a hypoglycemic who has gone without food for only a few hours.

If a migraine sufferer participates in a strenuous physical activity that burns up a considerable amount of glucose, it is very likely that his blood sugar will rapidly drop to below the level at which an attack is triggered. To prevent this from happening, the only solution is to supply the patient with an adequate amount of food immediately. A glass of orange juice followed by three or four crackers and, if possible, a piece of cheese would be enough.

A similar circumstance is encountered when a migraine patient suffers from severe emotional stress. This, as we know, can stimulate the pancreas to increase its production of insulin. During such periods the patient should be very careful to eat frequent meals that are rich in natural carbohydrates and completely devoid of sugar.

Heredity

Some persons can eat large amounts of processed sugars without the danger of becoming hypoglycemic or diabetic, while others cannot consume even small quantities without harming themselves. This different reaction of different individuals is not uncommon in human situations. If, for example, a group of individuals is fed exclusively white rice over a period of time, not all of them will contract beriberi. Of those who do, some will show only slight symptoms, while others will be seriously ill. Similarly, if a group of persons constantly receives an excess of sugar, as so often occurs in our modern world, the pancreas of some of them will continue to function correctly. In others this constant stimulus of excess sugar will disturb the normal functioning of the pancreas, producing excess insulin; this then alters the glucose equilibrium in the body, and these persons become hypoglycemics. In yet another group of people, the pancreas will exhaust itself and lose its capacity to secrete sufficient insulin, and the glucose equilibrium will be disturbed for a different reason; these persons will become diabetics.

These different reactions to the constant stimulus of excessive amounts of sugar depend on many variables. Both hypoglycemia and diabetes have a tendency to recur in the same family. In a study by A. P. Friedman and others of

564 patients suffering from migraine headaches, it was found that 46 percent of those patients suffering from common migraine and 40 percent of those with classical* migraine had a family history of headache in one or more close relatives. It has also been proved that the influence of the mother is much more frequent than that of the father, approximately in the ratio of two and a half cases to one.

Environment also predetermines in a sense whether or not an individual with the tendency for the disease will contract it. Hyperinsulinism appears to occur less in countries where meals are high in protein and natural carbohydrates and where there is a low per capita consumption of sugar. In poorer countries, where the diet of low-income families contains almost no protein, and in countries where refined-sugar consumption is high, the incidence of the disease is more common.

Do Diabetics Get Migraines?

It is obvious that if migraine is a consequence of low blood sugar and diabetes is the opposite affliction—that is, a disease in which there is too much sugar in the bloodstream—diabetics cannot suffer from migraine headache. As a matter of fact, over fifty years ago P. A. Gray and H. L. Burtness published a paper in the scientific journal *Endocrinology* stating that they had observed only four cases of migraine, or 0.9 percent, among 433 diabetics. I personally have known several hundred diabetics and very few of them had occa-

---

*Some authors separate migraine into classical and common (or ordinary). *Classical* is the name given to the headache preceded by neurological auras, such as scotomas; *common migraine* is the name given to the kind unaccompanied by preheadache phenomena. However, all types of migraine are the result of hyperinsulinism.

sional migraine attacks. The migraines occurred when they used an overdose of insulin or one of the synthetic hypoglycemic drugs and when for any other reason, such as the omission of a meal, their blood sugar level fell substantially below normal.

Can Continuous Doses of Glucose Avert Migraine Attacks?

Several papers were published during the 1930s that recommended diets rich in all kinds of carbohydrates for the prevention of migraine attacks. Moreover, some authors even prescribed massive doses of glucose or ordinary table sugar to alleviate them. We now know that their reasoning was incorrect; however, it is easy to see how they may have been led to this conclusion.

We have seen that when an individual eats sugar, the initial result is a hyperglycemia, or rise in the blood sugar. After a certain period of time, the pancreas of those predisposed to migraine produces an excessive quantity of insulin. This then leads to the hypoglycemia, which in turn causes a migraine attack. But what would happen if the individual were given an additional dose of glucose before the blood sugar level dropped below normal? Obviously the blood glucose would rise once again, thereby counteracting the incipient hypoglycemia and thus preventing the migraine attack from occurring. If sugar is given at regular intervals, so that the blood sugar level never falls below the normal range, the patient will never have an attack of migraine. It sounds like a perfectly easy and enjoyable solution, doesn't it? Well, don't get too excited yet.

I have had the opportunity to interview numerous patients for whom this treatment had been prescribed. Most of those who followed this advice found that they soon began to experience an acute pain in the area of the abdomen where the pancreas is located. The pain in question is the result of the increased demands that are being made on this organ. If the treatment were continued after the pain appeared, the pancreas might become so damaged that it would cease to produce even a sufficient amount of insulin, and the patient would become a diabetic. I have actually seen this happen in some migraine sufferers.

Chocolate

Most migraine patients have probably become aware that an attack can frequently be triggered by eating chocolate. This is usually misinterpreted as an allergic reaction to chocolate. However, it is interesting that dietetic chocolate, artificially sweetened with products other than sugar, does not produce migraine attacks in predisposed persons. This can easily be explained as follows.

The main components of chocolate are ground cacao seeds and sugar. The first of these components has by itself only a very slight hypoglycemic effect, not sufficient to trigger a migraine attack. However, when sugar is added to it, the hypoglycemic effects of both ingredients strongly reinforce one another, yielding one of the most powerful hypoglycemic combinations known. Migraine sufferers therefore must absolutely avoid this confection.

Other Refined Sugars

In addition to refined cane or beet sugar, which is almost 100 percent pure sucrose, foods may contain other refined sugars that are as detrimental to the health as sucrose because they also are almost 100 percent pure. The most frequently found are: glucose, also known as dextrose; fructose, synonymous with levulose; and corn syrup. By no means can a migraine sufferer eat any food containing these sugars.

Artificial Sweeteners

Some artificial sweeteners contain one of the above-mentioned sugars, and if foods or beverages are sweetened with one of them, the effect will be the same as that of ordinary sugar, which means that a migraine can be triggered.

Saccharin does not stimulate the pancreas to produce insulin and therefore does not have any influence on migraine headache, but saccharin may be hazardous to the health on other grounds—it has been determined to cause cancer in laboratory animals.

The newest artifical sweetener, widely used at the present time, is not a carbohydrate but an amino acid. This sweetener, which is a mixture of aspartic acid and the methyl ester of phenylalanin, has only a slight stimulating effect on the pancreas and is therefore usually harmless for most migraine sufferers if ingested in modest amounts.

11

How Do You Know?

Many years ago I enjoyed the experience of lecturing a group of medical students in general chemistry when their regular professor was forced, because of health problems, to take a leave of absence. During the term of my temporary assignment, many of the students became quite good friends of mine and I still correspond with some of them on a fairly regular basis. My rapport with the faculty of the medical school was also amicable and I can count several friends among that esteemed group as well.

When my research on migraine began to show positive results, I was quite naturally anxious to share my findings with my associates in the medical profession. Most of my old friends received my ideas with enthusiasm; however, not all of them were easily convinced. New ideas in medicine sometimes take many years to be totally accepted by the physicians who must practice them, and so I was not discouraged by the misgivings of some of my colleagues. I remember that Dr. Richard Bell, a professor in the medical school and a specialist in internal medicine, frequently came to see me at the lab, but our social visits usually ended in an argument over the validity of my work with migraine. He was of the opinion that I was completely on the wrong track and that migraine is an emotional, not a biochemical, disorder. Dr. Bell tried his best to convince me of my "error."

"Why do you insist that the disorder is a result of a faulty body chemistry only?" he used to argue. "Everyone knows that migraines are brought on by emotional conflicts. I am positive that it is simply coincidental that some of your patients have low blood sugar as well as migraine."

I tried many times to prove my theory to him with the great volume of experimental data I had collected over the years; however, because of his busy schedule he never had the time to listen. Perhaps, too, he was so totally convinced that he was right, he thought it a waste of time to hear me out.

Dr. Bell is a very intelligent man, one of the best professors at the medical school and a highly skilled physician as well. I have known him for many years and have great respect for him, as do many of his fellow doctors, his students, and his patients. His diagnoses have been known to be brilliant, and the lecture hall is filled to capacity when he conducts a class. Because of this, I suppose, I was more determined to persuade him than anyone else that my findings were correct. This was not easy since neither one of us seemed ever to have the time for a thorough discussion of the subject. When he visited my lab it was usually during the day when I was always busy with tests and evaluations. Whenever I had an opportunity to drop in on him, he was always occupied and could not talk for any length of time.

One day I changed my strategy and went to his office late in the afternoon, hoping for a longer visit. He had his coat on when I arrived, however, and was about to leave for home.

"Rudy," he said, "if you're not busy, why don't you come home with me for a drink? We are not likely to be interrupted there. Maybe we can finally have our talk. I relish the opportunity to disprove your migraine/low blood sugar theory," he chided me. "Why not give me a chance to change your mind?"

"Okay, Dick, I accept your challenge," I replied. "I am just as sure that I can convince you, my friend, of the opposite." And so we started the thirty-minute drive to his home.

"Did I ever tell you," he offered during the ride, "that my wife, Eleanor, has suffered from migraine since before we were married? No one, not the finest neurologists in the country, has been able to help her. She has recently put herself under the care of a psychiatrist and I am convinced that we have finally been pointed in the right direction. We'll be seeing some results soon, I'm sure."

I shook my head and laughed.

"You're a hard man to change, aren't you?" he chided.

When we arrived at their home, Eleanor greeted us at the door.

"How have you been, Professor Low? I haven't seen you for quite some time. But Dick talks about you often. You're looking well."

"Thank you, I am feeling good, but please call me Rudy. You're looking well yourself, Eleanor. How have you been?"

Eleanor was a pretty woman, although a bit overweight. I knew that she was about fifty years old, but she certainly didn't look it. I hadn't seen her for several years, but I immediately remembered her soft, pleasant voice and her lovely, unchanged face.

"Oh, I'm healthy enough, I guess," she answered.

"Everything would be perfect if it weren't for these damned headaches. I suppose Dick has told you about them. I know that I have to live with them, but sometimes I get desperate. I'm just so tired of waiting for another one to occur. It certainly ruins one's social life." She then stopped and excused herself. "Oh, listen to me. You haven't been here five minutes and all I've talked about is bad news. Come and sit down."

"I don't mind at all, Eleanor. You know, I have been into migraine research for over fifteen years and all of my patients—that's what I call them—have been completely relieved. Hasn't Dick told you?"

"No, I haven't," Dick interjected emphatically, "because I don't believe it!" He brought over a double scotch for Eleanor and began to prepare one for himself.

"Rudy, what will it be?"

"Dick, you wouldn't by any chance have any unsweetened fruit juice in the house, would you?"

He laughed. "You never give up, do you, Rudy? Believe me, a jigger of scotch will do you more good than the juice, but if you insist . . . Eleanor, don't we have some fresh orange juice?"

His wife left and returned with a tall icy glass of juice. She also offered me some cheese and crackers, which I gladly accepted.

"Dick, I thought that you were going to allow me to present my case. Would you mind if I ask your wife some questions about her migraines for a start?"

"Go right ahead, if Eleanor doesn't mind. This should be interesting." He sat back in his easy chair and sipped his drink.

"Eleanor," I said, "would you mind very much answering some boring questions?"

"I would do anything, even if there was only a slight chance that my migraines could be relieved."

"Your chances are not as remote as you may think. I can assure you of that," I said, looking in Dick's direction. I then began to ask Eleanor the same questions that I ask all my patients when I see them for the first time.

"Eleanor, when did your trouble begin?"

"My attacks began when I was thirteen, but then they were not as frequent as they are now. They used to occur only every month or so."

"Please, if you will, describe the pain you feel. Does your whole head hurt, or is the pain more intense on one side than the other?"

"Oh, the pain is almost always on the right side of my head."

"Is it a throbbing type of pain?"

"Yes, that's it exactly."

"Before the actual pain begins, do you have any visual disturbances such as the ability to see only half of all objects? Dick would call this hemianopsia."

"Oh, yes, all of my migraines begin in this way."

"Afterward, I bet you see spots of different colors swirling before your eyes. They're called scintillating scotomas."

"I see the spots all right, but mine aren't in technicolor," she laughed. "I'm afraid I'm only blessed with the black-and-white variety."

"Do you lose the feeling on one side of your face or in your tongue and fingers?"

"I do in most instances, but not always."

"Where does this loss of feeling occur?"

"Let me see, usually in my hand on the side where the headache is."

"Do you experience nausea during your attacks?"

"Always, much to my regret. I hate that feeling."

"Do you vomit?"

"Never. I guess I try to hold it back. As I've said, I dislike being nauseous, and vomiting is horrible as far as I'm concerned. When I was a girl I did get sick a few times during my attacks, but I don't anymore."

"Have you ever experienced amnesia at the height of an attack?"

"It did happen several times, though I wouldn't exactly call it amnesia. You see, I get mixed up and can't even remember the names of my children, and sometimes not my own. It sounds so ridiculous, doesn't it? And yet when it happens it's always very frightening. Sometimes during an attack I have a difficult time expressing myself."

"Eleanor, everything that you have told me is a characteristic of severe migraine. Of course, other diseases can produce a similar type of headache with symptoms such as yours. An intracranial tumor, for instance, is one such disorder; however, we can definitely rule this out in your case since your attacks have lasted for thirty-seven years. Now, Eleanor, I would very much like to know the kinds of food that you eat. I know this is a very personal question, but I must know if we are to prevent your migraines. Would you mind very much telling me?"

"No, I don't think so, Rudy."

"Okay, good. I'm interested in everything that you put into your stomach, from breakfast until bedtime. Oh, and also don't forget to include snacks."

"Well, as you can see, Rudy, I'm overweight and I'm very conscious of it. I try to cut down at breakfast by having just a cup of coffee without cream and sometimes a piece of toast."

"Do you put sugar into your coffee?"

"Unfortunately, yes. I just can't drink my coffee completely black."

"Eleanor, it would be better for you to use cream and leave out the sugar if you must have coffee. Go on."

"Well, for lunch I eat what everyone else does these days. I might have a sandwich or a piece of pizza, but sometimes I'm content with only a fruit salad."

"What? No dessert, no drink like coffee or tea?"

"Oh, yes, I have to confess that I like a sweet after a meal. I'm sure that you've guessed that already by my size," she answered sheepishly. "I keep ice cream bars in the freezer for my grandchildren and I've been eating them lately. Sometimes I nibble at cookies as well. If it's a hot day I usually drink a Coke with my lunch, but if it's cool I have hot coffee instead."

"With sugar, of course?"

"Well, yes, what's wrong with that? Doesn't just about everyone use sugar in their coffee?" I just smiled and so she continued. "For dinner we have the usual meal, either beef or chicken and occasionally fish. We usually accompany this with a salad and one or two vegetables. Believe me, Rudy, it's well balanced, if that's what you're getting at. Sometimes we follow up with a dessert, but not always."

"Tell me, Eleanor, don't you have any snacks between meals?"

"Now you've hit a sensitive spot, Rudy."

"Well, if you'd rather not answer . . ."

"Oh, I guess it doesn't matter that much. Naturally I have snacks. I really have a passion for sweets—cookies, pies, doughnuts, you know, everything that ruins your figure. I used to eat chocolate, but I've been trying to avoid it lately. It doesn't seem to agree with me."

"In what way?"

"Oh, I don't know. It seems to me that I always get one of my migraines after I eat chocolate. Does that sound silly?"

"Not at all. I'm sorry about all of the questions, but I really would like to help you. Do you take any medicines?"

Dick went to make himself another drink and mumbled something about talking to the walls.

"I usually take just plain aspirin for my headaches, not that it does any good. I sometimes also take a sleeping pill at night. Dick prescribed this for me. You see, I'm a very high-strung person." She showed me her medicine bottle; it was a nitrobenzodiazepine derivative. (As explained in Chapter 8, this is a pancreatic stimulator.)

"What about alcohol?"

"We usually have a scotch or two before dinner, and sometimes an after-dinner drink."

"For heaven's sake, Dick," I almost yelled. "After what I've just heard, it's no wonder that your wife gets migraines!"

"Rudy, I don't see what this all proves. Eleanor's diet is no different from anyone else's."

I then, for once without any interruptions, explained to Dr. Bell my theory on migraine. I told him that the high insulin secretion by his wife's overactive pancreas caused the counterregulatory mechanism of her body to be activated. The catecholamines were produced and a migraine thus initiated. I also told him that many products, especially but not only refined sugar, can stimulate the production of an abnormally high amount of insulin in individuals whose pancreas is overactive, and explained how the attacks can be prevented by an appropriate diet.

"But, Rudy, how do you know that the pancreas of a migraine patient produces too much insulin?"

"Dick, I have actually measured insulin secretions in both healthy individuals and migraine sufferers and found quite different results in the two groups. The secretion of insulin in migraine patients is usually much faster than in normal persons and reaches higher values, while the return to the initial level is sometimes delayed. Furthermore, the insulin curves of a high percentage of migraine sufferers show a special pattern in which the concentration of insulin reaches a maximum, then goes down, and, without any new stimulation, climbs again to a second maximum. In other words, the insulin curve has two peaks instead of one. In some instances there are even three peaks. Just a moment—I have some charts in my briefcase that you might find interesting. You see," I said with a grin, "I came prepared. This one [see Figure 12] shows the variation of the concentration of insulin in the blood plasma of an actual migraine patient after the ingestion of one hundred grams of glucose. As you can see, the concentration of insulin rises very fast, then falls to almost the fasting value, and again goes up without any additional stimulation.

"This other chart [see Figure 13] shows the insulin concentrations in the blood plasma of another actual patient, who suffered from extremely severe migraine headaches.

"As a contrast to these figures, look at *this* chart [see Figure 14], where I have plotted the average insulin values of ten completely healthy young individuals against time. As you will notice, the rise of the insulin values is not as fast here as in the case of the migraine patients, and the peak of the curve is lower.

"It is important to know that the actual amount of insulin produced does not only depend on the highest point of the curve, but is measured by the whole area between the curve and the horizontal axis. I could show you many insulin curves of migraine patients and you would notice that in most of them this area is much greater than in normal individuals."

"I have to admit, Rudy, that this is very convincing data.

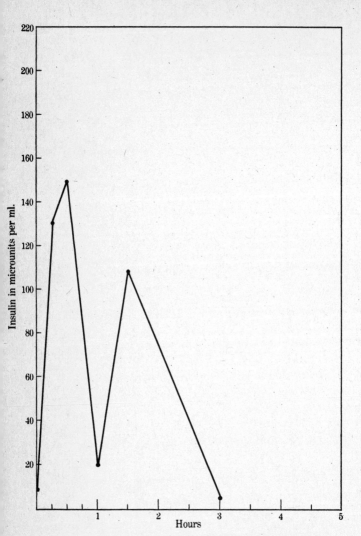

Figure 12. *Variation of the concentration of insulin in the blood plasma of migraine patient G.H. after the ingestion of 100 grams of glucose.*

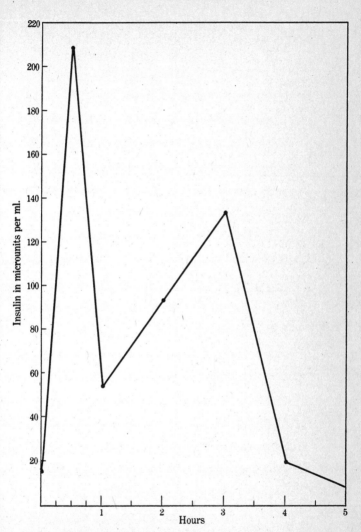

Figure 13. *Variation of the concentration of insulin in the blood plasma of migraine patient M.M. after the ingestion of 100 grams of glucose.*

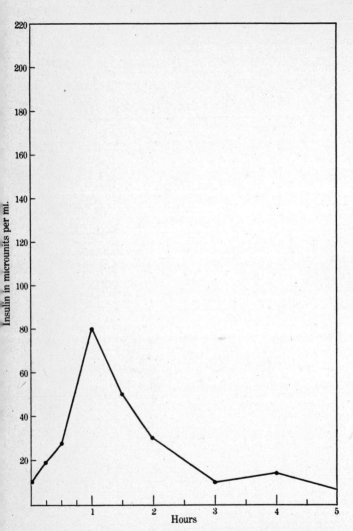

Figure 14. *Average variation of the concentration of insulin in the blood plasma of ten completely healthy young individuals.*

Nothing of this sort has been previously published, has it?"

"This is all my own research, Dick. It was published in several papers some time ago."*

"Well, Eleanor, why not give it a try? Rudy, what is the exact treatment that you have worked out?"

"First and foremost, Eleanor, you must completely give up refined sugar and all products that contain it. You have seen how sugar stimulates the pancreas of migraine sufferers to produce a large amount of insulin. This is the first step in the making of a migraine and so refined sugar must be avoided. Second, you'll have to eat at least six times a day because your pancreas is so active that even without the stimulation of sugar, enough insulin is produced to bring on an attack."

"What would such a diet be like?" Eleanor inquired.

"Let me give you an example of what you might eat on a given day: unsweetened orange juice, ham or eggs, one to two pieces of toast and light coffee without sugar for breakfast; a small cheese sandwich at midmorning; spaghetti and meatballs and light coffee for lunch; a chunk of cheese and some crackers at midafternoon; sirloin steak with french fries, a lettuce and tomato salad, and an apple for dinner; and finally some crackers before you go to bed."

"But, Rudy, I am already overweight and I will get even heavier on a diet such as this!"

"No, you won't, Eleanor. I give you my personal guarantee."

"Yes, she will," interrupted Dick. "She will be eating at least twice as much as she usually does."

"That may be so, but this diet does not contain any refined sugar and therefore she will not gain any weight. On the contrary, she will probably lose some. Furthermore, if she

*See references under Low in the Bibliography.

reduces only slightly the amount of starchy foods, such as bread, crackers, and potatoes, in my recommended diet, she will in fact lose several pounds."

"Well, Eleanor," said Dick, who was still not completely convinced, "I suppose it wouldn't hurt to give it a try."

Eleanor was much more enthusiastic than her husband. "Of course I'll do it," she exclaimed.

I gave Eleanor Bell an example of a diet for a migraine patient and cautioned that she must also abstain from alcohol.

"Later, once you have completely recovered, you can try small amounts of table wine now and then. However, you must never drink any sweet wine or hard liquor or beer."

"That shouldn't be any problem for me," she said. "I'm not really that fond of alcohol."

"Oh, and Dick," I said. "Please, you must withdraw the sleeping pills that you prescribed for your wife."

"Are you telling me what medicines to give my own wife?" he retorted indignantly.

"I'm sorry, Dick, but she will not get rid of her headaches if she continues on this medicine, even if she adheres to her diet. It is poison to a hypoglycemic; it is a nitrobenzodiazepine derivative, a drug that can stimulate the pancreas. She must also stop taking aspirin since this, too, is hypoglycemic in nature.

"To prove my point, let me do a determination of the insulin concentration in Eleanor's blood plasma after one of her usual sugar-rich meals followed by two aspirins. I'll make you a wager that the results will be at least twice the normal value."

"Okay, you're on, that is if Eleanor doesn't mind. After all, it is her body we're talking about."

Eleanor approved the test and several days later I showed Dick the results. The insulin determination, performed after her meal and medication, showed a rise in the insulin concentration to almost 300 microcounts per milliliter of blood plasma in only a few minutes. Dr. Bell was at last a convert.

Eleanor had a few tough days in the beginning, but one and a half months after the start of her therapy she no longer needed any of her medicines. Now, after thirty-seven years of pain and misery, she has completely recovered. In addition, she has lost twenty pounds and looks even younger than she did on the day when I first explained my theory to her. Her husband, Dr. Bell, has since given several speeches supporting my work and always includes his wife's recovery as an example of how migraine can be eliminated through diet therapy.

12

Treatment

It is not an exaggeration to say that on the average there are about twenty hypoglycemics among every one hundred individuals. In the great majority of these cases hyperinsulinism, the excessive secretion of insulin by the pancreas, is the cause of the disorder. The incidence of hypoglycemia has increased considerably as a result of our modern, sugar-rich diets that overwork the pancreas. About 40 to 50 percent of all hypoglycemics also suffer from migraine along with their other discomforts. By now it must be clear to the reader that the various manifestations of hypoglycemia, including migraine, disappear when the patient avoids all refined sugars and follows the other easy recommendations set forth in this book. This solution to the age-old problem of migraine may seem almost too simple for such a severe and previously mysterious disease. Nevertheless, the treatment has proved itself to be completely effective: over 90 percent of the migraine patients who followed it have been completely relieved of their attacks. The treatment, which will bring the migraine sufferer new health and a life that is free from the pain of migraine, is presented below in the form of four rules. Before reading them, however, you must know that headaches can be produced by a great variety of causes, ranging from a common cold to a life-threatening brain tumor. It is therefore necessary to have an unquestionable diagnosis of migraine headache from a medical doctor; only then can these rules be implemented.

Rule Number One

The first rule of migraine treatment is: *Completely eliminate refined sugar from the diet.* Whether added directly to coffee, tea, or cereal as a sweetener, or eaten as an ingredient of foods such as cakes, candies, chocolates, canned fruits, cookies, custards, dried fruits, fruit-flavored yogurt, ice cream, jams, soft drinks, or sweet liqueurs and wines, all refined sugars, not only sucrose but also glucose, fructose, and corn syrup, must be avoided. Many prepared foods, mentioned in Chapter 13, contain sugar although they don't appear sweet, and they must be avoided as well. The migraine patient must exchange a diet rich in refined sugar for one that is high in natural sugars and carbohydrates, such as fruits, potatoes, rice, and wheat flour, and that has adequate protein. For modern man, hooked on the sugar habit, this involves a self-retraining process. The migraine patient will have to develop new eating habits, and may even learn to like them better than his old ones.

It is extremely important that every person subject to migraine find out, before eating or drinking anything, whether the food or beverage in question contains any refined sugars; if it does, he must strictly avoid it. This fundamental rule of the treatment must be observed rigorously, since *even seemingly insignificant amounts of sugar can trigger attacks of incredible severity*. This rule must also be followed continuously; if after a time the person goes back to eating sugar, the symptoms will reappear.

Many patients feel that it is too difficult to eliminate all foods containing refined sugar from their diet and prefer instead to continue suffering from the ailment. Of course, it all depends on how severe the problem is. If a person's migraine is limited to a headache that can be controlled by common painkillers, he may choose to put up with the discomfort and take the medications when necessary, rather than deprive himself of the foods he most enjoys. But for the person who suffers from an incapacitating type of migraine, any sacrifice will seem small in comparison to the relief he will experience. It will not be too hard for him to completely eliminate those foods that precipitate his attacks of migraine.

In our culture it can sometimes be difficult to eliminate refined sugar. Whether in North America, South America, Europe, or the Orient, breakfast usually includes a cup of tea or coffee with milk, sweetened with from one to three teaspoonsful of sugar (about 5 to 15 grams), often accompanied by a sweet roll, Danish pastry, or doughnut, each containing a large quantity of sugar. It is common to start the day with a cereal that is already inherently high in sugar and then dump more into it. Some people even have one of the many sugary orange drinks that attempt to pass for the real thing. These orange-juice impostors must even be supplemented by the addition of vitamin C for them to claim any significant nutritional value. How ironic that the manufacturers deliberately destroy the natural vitamins contained in a foodstuff, then turn around and add the synthetic variety and call their product "vitamin enriched," leading the consumer to believe he is actually getting additional nutrients.

If a healthy individual eats a breakfast like the one just described, chances are that he will at least feel perfectly well, although the possibility does exist that this constant stimulus to his pancreas may ultimately result in hypoglycemia. However, for an individual already suffering from this condition (whether he is aware of it or not), the large quantity of sugar consumed at such a meal will force his pancreas to release excessive amounts of insulin. He will leave home each day in a veritable state of shock, like a diabetic who has received an overdose of insulin. This may explain why many people start the day nervous, tired, and in bad temper.

But this is only the beginning of the day. There are few people who do *not* have a soft drink (approximately 20 grams of sugar) or a cup of coffee or tea with sugar in the midmorning, and if they are hungry even a pastry, cookies, or some other sweet as well. This is especially true in the case of a hypoglycemic since, if he has eaten the breakfast described above, his pancreas will have produced so much insulin that the desire for something sweet will be overwhelming.

Lunch and dinner provide no relief, either, from our "sugarmania." Most of us include a soft drink or other sweetened beverage with our meals, and it has become a nearly universal custom to finish lunch and dinner with a dessert—usually pie, cake, ice cream, or canned fruit.

Even more common these days is to skip lunch altogether and head right for the dessert. And if this were not enough, some people feel they cannot go to bed without a snack of cookies, a soft drink, ice cream, or another pastry or sweet, thus providing a final blow to their much-abused pancreas.

And yet, despite all of this, we continue to express surprise at the number of diabetics and hypoglycemics; the real wonder is that there are not many more!

A migraine patient now knows what *not* to eat, but what kinds of foods should be in his diet? The first step is to start the day with a good breakfast, since without this the brain will be in a state of starvation during the hours when it is usually required to work the hardest. The habit of omitting this meal, which some people have cultivated, frequently is the precipitating factor in their precarious state of health. An ideal breakfast should contain a fruit, preferably but not necessarily a glass of unsweetened orange juice, and a natural carbohydrate, such as one to two pieces of toast, or an equivalent amount of bread, crackers, or cereal. It is also advisable to supplement the protein contained in the above with a protein-rich food, such as cheese, or a small piece of meat or chicken left over from the day before, or occasionally with a slice of ham or an egg. At first glance, this new way of life might seem to be a hardship to the time-conscious, intemperate, modern individual. However, for those who have suffered from the symptoms of migraine, developing these new habits will not be difficult when they begin to experience, probably for the first time in years, complete and lasting health in mind and body.

Lunch for the migraine patient should include a generous portion of meat, fish, or poultry and one or two vegetables, especially starchy ones such as potatoes. For example, a midday meal could consist of chicken prepared in the desired manner, with broccoli in cheese sauce and a baked potato. This same meal could be eaten with a salad; in this case the dressing must be sugar-free. For dessert, if desired, fresh fruit would be perfect. Since many of us who are plagued with migraine are members of the busy working community and are often limited at noon to one hour or less for our meal, less time-consuming suggestions for lunch will be given in a special cookbook now in preparation.

Similarly, the evening meal should consist of meat, fish, or poultry with a natural carbohydrate and vegetables. Rigidity of nutritional requirements need not limit the imagination. The old saying that "variety is the spice of life" can also be applied to the diet of the hypoglycemic. Learn to alternate different types of meat, fish, poultry, and eggs with new and novel carbohydrate and vegetable recipes.

The main dish in all the meals eaten by the migraine patient should always be rich in natural carbohydrates (potatoes, rice, pasta, etc.) and should also contain a high-protein food. Ideal sources of the latter are meat, fish, poultry, eggs, and cheese. Many people have never even tried meats such as heart, lungs, kidney, brains, and liver. As a rule, these are less expensive then other, more popular cuts and have superior nutritional value. This is especially true of liver. Meats other than beef are likewise looked upon with disdain and are unappreciated. Goat, lamb, rabbit, and venison are high in nutritional value and, when well prepared, have an excellent taste. Pork and ham also have a high nutritional value, but cuts with too much fat are hard to digest for some people. Vegetables are essential components of any diet and must be eaten by the migraine sufferer as well. There are a great variety of vegetables from which to choose:

artichokes	cabbage (raw and cooked)
asparagus	carrots
beans (other than kidney and lima beans)	cauliflower
beets	celery (raw and cooked)
broccoli	chard leaves
Brussels sprouts	chick-peas
	corn

cucumbers	pepper, green
eggplant	potatoes
kohlrabi	pumpkin
lentils	radishes
lettuce	spinach
mushrooms	squash
okra	tomatoes
onions	turnip greens
peas	turnips

Notice that both lima beans and kidney beans are excluded. The reason is that, like fatty meats such as pork, they are often difficult to digest. Undigested food may undergo fermentation in the intestine, thereby producing substances that have hypoglycemic effects—substances capable of stimulating the pancreas to produce insulin.

There are many books available that suggest specific diets for the hypoglycemic. Most of them, however, include a basic mistake: they fail to make clear the difference between "refined sugar" and "processed carbohydrate." Ordinary sugar, or sucrose, is a carbohydrate that is almost 100 percent pure—making it a very harmful disaccharide. White wheat flour, on the other hand, still contains other natural ingredients needed for its correct metabolism in the body; thus it is not a chemically pure polysaccharide. A migraine patient, therefore, can eat large amounts of foods made with flour, as long as they do not contain sugar. Chemically pure starch is as harmful as pure sugar; however, it is only a laboratory curiosity—we are unlikely to encounter it. Most literature on the treatment of hypoglycemia recommends limiting the intake of all carbohydrates, whether they are chemically pure or in their natural state. I emphasize that natural carbohydrates are, on the contrary, absolutely necessary for hypoglycemic individuals, whose principal source of glucose is provided by the hydrolysis of the starch contained in them. Hypoglycemics actually need carbohydrates more than healthy individuals do; but these carbohydrates must be natural. A hypoglycemic absolutely cannot tolerate refined sugars.

Finally, an important remark. *Fruits must always be eaten fresh, never dried, cooked, or baked, because some of the components provided by nature that are needed for the correct utilization of sugars by the body are destroyed when fruits are dried, cooked, or baked.*

Rule Number Two

The second rule of migraine treatment, as important as the first, is: *Never allow more than two to three hours to go by without eating.* The pancreas of migraine sufferers is so highly overactive that approximately two hours after a meal the level of insulin in the blood begins to go above normal even without the stimulation of refined sugar. At three hours the level is usually high enough to initiate a migraine attack. However, if the patient eats something at that time, especially if he eats a natural carbohydrate, the insulin will be used up and the attack will not take place. Therefore it is essential for the migraine patient to give up the habit, so strongly ingrained in us, of eating only three meals a day. Instead, he should establish the custom of eating *at least* six times daily: at breakfast, midmorning, noon, midafternoon, in the evening, and before going to bed.

By no means should the interval between meals exceed three hours. If this time interval is exceeded, a migraine attack is very likely. To avoid such an event, it is important always to carry some food in the pocket or in the purse.

For most migraine sufferers six meals, three average and three small, are sufficient, provided that the three-hour interval is not exceeded. In severe cases, however, even this may be inadequate; and more than one small meal or snack between breakfast and lunch or between lunch and dinner may be required. Intervals of two hours are usually adequate in such cases.

During sleep, the activity of the pancreas decreases substantially, so it is usually not necessary to break this long fast. However, in exceptional cases the migraine victim would benefit by taking some nourishment in the middle of the night.

A good midmorning snack—or midafternoon and bedtime snack—would be two or three handfuls of peanuts or cashews, or a few crackers, or a small cheese or ham sandwich. There are many ways to vary this small meal, but its principal component must be a food rich in natural carbohydrates.

Experience has shown that, in order to maintain the correct nutritional equilibrium of the body, the elimination of refined sugar must be counterbalanced by an *increased amount of natural carbohydrates*, more or less in the ratio by weight of one part sugar to two and a half parts natural carbohydrates. The recommended ratio is only approximate and by no means are you required to weigh your foods. There is a much simpler way to find out if you are ingesting the correct amount of natural carbohydrates: Once a week check your weight on a scale. If you are losing weight, you must eat more natural carbohydrates; if you are gaining weight, you must eat less. This is an easy and most effective method.

One further important point: *Fruits should always be eaten with the main meal, never alone or as a snack.* As explained above, the concentration of insulin in the blood of a migraine sufferer is higher than normal for some time after eating. If at that time he eats a fruit, the danger exists that even the very slight stimulating effect of the fruit may bring the total amount of insulin to the critical point at which a migraine attack is triggered.

Rule Number Three

It has been proved by many scientific studies that the ingestion of alcohol is one of the most frequent causes of hypoglycemia. This hypoglycemia is due not to an abnormally strong stimulation of the pancreas, but rather to the inhibition of the glycogenic function of the liver—that is, its ability to store glycogen and to release glucose. Consequently, we have the third rule of migraine treatment: *Avoid alcoholic beverages, especially the most concentrated ones.* Sweet wines and liqueurs, as we have mentioned, almost always precipitate migraine attacks in predisposed individuals, due to the combined action of two hypoglycemic substances: alcohol and sugar. As explained in Chapter 8, beer is especially harmful, due to the combined action of three hypoglycemic components: maltose, alcohol, and oxalic acid.

Rule Number Four

The fourth rule of migraine treatment is: *Avoid hypoglycemia-producing drugs.* If the patient is taking only aspirin for the pain of the migraine, he will soon be able to do without it if he follows the prescribed diet. If, however, he is taking other medicines to control other ailments while following the prescribed diet and is still not experiencing any relief, then one of these drugs must be at fault. He should then discuss this condition with his doctor, who will decide whether he can stop taking the drug or, if this is not possible, whether he can replace it with another one of equivalent pharmacological value but without hypoglycemic effects.

In connection with this rule, it should also be remembered that a large amount of caffeine can likewise trigger an attack. Patients who suffer from migraines must therefore avoid the consumption of too much strong coffee and tea, and some of the popular soft drinks that contain caffeine. Beverages that contain both caffeine and sugar are especially to be avoided.

In summary, *migraine attacks can be prevented in over 90 percent of all cases with a diet of six or more meals daily that are rich in natural carbohydrates, adequate in protein, and completely devoid of processed sugars and alcoholic beverages, provided that all kinds of drugs with hypoglycemic effects, as well as an excess of caffeine, are also omitted.*

This is obviously a harmless diet. However, a migraine patient might also suffer from another ailment that requires a different diet. It is therefore recommended that he discuss his condition with his doctor before initiating the treatment.

The time required to get rid of migraine headache depends on several conditions, including the intensity of the symptoms, the time passed since the initiation of the attacks, and the age of the patient. Young persons whose symptoms have lasted no more than a few years and are relatively mild usually recover in less than one month, while older persons who have suffered severe symptoms for many years may require several months to recover completely. The average time required is usually between one and two months. In most cases the symptoms begin to subside soon after the start of the regimen. However, occasionally, at the beginning of the treatment there is some worsening while the body adjusts to the new regimen. It is imperative that the patient know this and is encouraged to continue following the rules in order to obtain complete relief.

Finally, if an error is made, for whatever reason, and even a small amount of sugar is eaten, a large quantity of water should be ingested immediately so that the sugar will reach the bloodstream in a less concentrated form. Its harmful effects on the pancreas will thereby be reduced. Do not, however, make the mistake of misinterpreting this as an antidote. It is *not* permissible to eat a small amount of sugar from time to time and afterward drink a large quantity of water. The above advice should be reserved only at those times when sugar is eaten inadvertently.

13

Label Reading

In order to avoid sugar, a migraine patient must be aware of all the ingredients that go into the products he consumes. This means careful reading of labels at the supermarket to identify "safe products," something that may take a little extra time at first, but that will be well worth the initial bother.

The following survey is intended only as a guide to get you started as an observant shopper who suffers from migraine. It was conducted in two large American supermarket chains only, which means that there probably are many more different types of acceptable products available to the public. Specialty- and health-food shops, for example, carry interesting alternatives to the more common commodities found in the larger stores. I want to emphasize that, although this survey includes a great number of products, it by no means covers every available foodstuff. It is up to you to locate safe products by reading labels.

Ingredients for a product are listed on the label according to their percentage by weight of the whole. The constituent that comes first on the label is the one that the total product contains the highest amount of, and so on through the entire list to the last and least ingredient. If, for instance, sugar is listed second, you can be sure that the item in question contains quite a large amount of it. You may be surprised to see how many "prepared" foods contain significant amounts of sugar.

Your new shopping habits should not substantially increase your food costs. Store brands are generally available to provide a choice other than the more expensive "name" brands. For instance, if an expensive brand of a product contains no added sugar, the less costly store brand is very likely to be available in this form also. You will find yourself buying more fresh fruits and vegetables. This may increase your food budget somewhat, since it appears that the less that is added to a commodity, the more it costs. It is ironic that unsweetened, natural fruit juice should be more expensive than the processed variety with added sugar. This increase, however, will probably be offset by the elimination from your shopping list of the high-priced convenience foods—not to mention candy and sweetened "junk" foods—since these as a rule contain some sucrose.

Cereals

Because of their convenience and availability, cereals are very good sources of natural carbohydrates. Unfortunately, cereals that do not contain refined sugar are very difficult to find. Some are obviously unacceptable since they are actually sugar-coated. The ingredients in most cereals will greatly surprise the consumer: most cereals, even the popular whole-wheat and high-protein varieties, contain large amounts of sugar. And the so-called health-food cereals that contain no artificial ingredients or white sugar are, nevertheless, sweetened with brown sugar and honey. The manufacturers of brown sugar would have us believe that because it is coarser and not as pretty as its pale relative, it is less refined. This is not true. Brown sugar is simply ordinary refined sugar dyed with molasses and therefore is just as harmful to the migraine sufferer as is white sugar.

Honey is a natural product and so we might conclude that it will not have any adverse effect on a migraine patient. However, a large amount of honey can trigger an attack. This is probably because of the presence of a small amount of a substance in honey commonly known as "royal jelly," which has a stimulating effect on the pancreas. In general, though, the amount of honey added to cereals is not enough to be of any harm. Thus, if a cereal contains only honey and no sugar, it can be consumed by the migraine patient without any problem.

Cereals that do not specifically mention sugar in their list of ingredients include Grape-Nuts (but not Grape-Nuts Flakes), shredded wheat, puffed rice, puffed wheat, Cream of Wheat, plain oatmeal, Quick Oats, Wheatena, and unflavored wheat germ. Instant grits have become a common dish to serve with breakfast in some parts of the country. Both the regular and bacon-flavored grits are sugar-free.

We have become so used to our sugar-rich cereals that the unsweetened ones listed above, if served only with milk, may seem unpalatable at first. The addition of fresh fruit will enhance their flavor, and you will soon learn to appreciate their true taste. Blueberries, strawberries, sliced peaches, and bananas are tasty and nutritious additions to any breakfast cereal.

Breads, Crackers, and Pasta

Although bread is one of the best sources of natural carbohydrates, it happens that many kinds, especially those for toasting, contain sugar, though others do not. You will probably have no problem in purchasing the bread you need to eat at home, but it is different if you eat out. Fortunately the bread used for sandwiches is sugar-free in most cases or contains only immeasurable amounts of sugar. My recommendation is to taste a little piece of it. If it contains sugar, you will notice it easily and you should not eat it.

Most whole-wheat breads are made not with sugar but with honey or molasses. Although an excessive intake of honey can be a threat to the migraine patient, there is not enough added to bread to have such an effect. An average loaf of whole-wheat bread contains only about one-quarter cup of honey, and this would likely be ingested over several days.

Molasses is also damaging to the migraine patient, though less so than white sugar. Some natural ingredients remain in the molasses, while others are destroyed or removed in the manufacturing process. Molasses, which is the syrup left after the sugar has crystallized out of the cane or beet juice, contains about 50 to 80 percent sugar. If a migraine patient eats whole-wheat bread and finds that he is not experiencing complete relief by following the treatment set forth in this book, it may well be that the molasses added to his bread is responsible. This, however, happens very seldom.

As for crackers, there are several varieties that do not list sugar as an ingredient. It is interesting that some brands of saltines are made with sugar while others, such as Nabisco and Keebler saltines, are not. Triscuits and RyKrisps are especially good since they are sugar-free and prepared with 100 percent whole-wheat flour. Sunshine Cheez-Its also do not list sugar as a constituent. Pretzels, on the other hand, are generally made with either corn syrup or sugar.

Macaroni and other types of pasta are excellent sources of carbohydrates for the migraine patient. All uncooked pasta is sugar-free, but beware of the canned types that are already in sauce or gravy. Most prepared foods, packaged in cans or jars, have a significant amount of sugar added and must be avoided. Homemade sauce for pasta is, as our mothers and grandmothers will tell us, simple to make and much tastier than the "ready-made" variety. Sugarfree canned all-purpose tomato sauces, tomato pastes and purees, as well as whole canned tomatoes are also available.

Fruits and Juices

Fresh fruits and fruit juices are rich in vitamins and natural sugar and should therefore be included in the diet of a migraine patient. Ideally these should be eaten only with other foods at mealtimes, not between meals. I strongly recommend that you eat your fruit "fresh from the market," since drying, stewing, or cooking it could have an adverse effect. Canned fruits are usually sweetened with either sugar or corn syrup, but if you look carefully you may also find them packed in water or in their own natural juices. Corn syrup, produced by hydrolysis of the starch contained in corn, is chemically composed largely of pure glucose. A product labeled "corn sweetened" has simply been sweetened with corn syrup and consequently must be eliminated from the diet. Applesauce, though usually made with sugar, is also available unsweetened.

Whether or not a juice is sweetened depends, it seems,

more on the type of fruit or vegetable that went into its making than on the brand. For example, most brands of apple juice, including the cheaper store brand, can be found without sugar. Cranberry juice, as well as the cranberry-apple variety, does have corn syrup added to it. In the "Low Cal" cranberry juices, the corn syrup is replaced with sodium saccharin.

Grapefruit juice is available in its natural state under most labels. This is also true of pineapple juice; however, odd as it may seem, pineapple-grapefruit juice usually contains additional sugar. Both peach and pear nectar can be found only with sugar, but grape juice is available both with and without sugar. There appears to be a rule of thumb where grape juice is concerned. If it is in a bottle and labeled "juice" then it is usually, but not always, sugar-free. Grape-ades and grape "drinks," usually found in cans, are not.

Tomato juices are usually flavored only with salt. However, when beef or clam flavoring is added, so too is sugar. The popular multivegetable juice contains no sugar.

A word of caution: Be careful of all fruit "drinks" and "punches." These are always high in sugar and must be eliminated from the diet of the migraine patient. Lemonade and frozen grape juice are also high in sugar, but unsweetened orange juice is available as a frozen concentrate or ready to drink in cartons and cans.

In conclusion, all of the nondietetic canned fruits surveyed for this book, with the exception of canned pineapple, contained sugar or corn syrup. Many fruit juices are available without sugar; however, one must search for them. Since there is an ever-increasing demand for natural products, in the near future the consumer will probably have more of a choice in his purchase of the popular brands of canned fruits and juices.

Vegetables

The sugar content of vegetables in cans also appears to be a function more of the particular product than of the brand. The following list of canned vegetables may serve as a guide for you. The vegetables have been divided into two categories: those that can be found without sugar and those that are usually sweetened with sugar. This does not mean that *all* brands of vegetables listed in the first column are sugar-free, nor that all brands of vegetables in the second column contain sugar. You yourself must check the labels to be absolutely sure.

Canned Vegetables

Sugar-Free	*With Sugar*
artichoke hearts	baked beans
asparagus	barbecued beans
beans with chili	butter beans
beets, sliced	corn, cream-style
black beans	corn, regular
carrots	French-fried onions
chick-peas	German potato salad
collard greens	Harvard beets
field peas with snaps	kidney beans
green beans	onions, whole
lima beans	peas
mixed vegetables	peas and carrots
mushrooms	pickled beets
mustard greens	pork and beans
northern beans	potato salad
okra	sauerkraut, Bavarian-style
potatoes, boiled	stewed tomatoes
sauerkraut, regular	three-bean salad
spinach	vegetable salad

Sugar-Free	*With Sugar*
tomatoes, whole	yams
tomato paste	zucchini
tomato puree	
turnip greens	
wax beans	
yellow squash	

Cornstarch and potato starch are excellent natural carbohydrates and are therefore among the safe products for the migraine patient. They are sometimes found in boxed instant potatoes, in soups, and in other foods as thickeners. Instant mashed potatoes, instant hash browns, and potato pancakes are usually free from sugar; instant scalloped potatoes, however, are not.

Many of the popular canned soups do not list sugar as an ingredient. Most brands of the following are in this category: chicken noodle, chicken vegetable, chunky beef, chunky chicken, chunky chicken with rice, chunky sirloin burger, cream of chicken, cream of mushroom, cream of potato, lentil, Manhattan clam chowder, minestrone, New England clam chowder, onion, turkey noodle, and vegetable beef. Plain split pea does contain dextrose, and the ham in split pea with ham is cured with dextrose. Most plain broths and bouillon cubes contain either dextrose or sugar and corn syrup.

Frozen Products

Frozen vegetables are excellent and closely approximate their fresh counterparts in nutritional value. All plain frozen vegetables, such as cut green beans or carrots not in sauce, are in their natural state and consequently free from refined sugar. It is the fancy sauces and seasonings that get you into trouble. Invariably, vegetables cooked in butter or with other sauces and seasonings are also flavored with sugar. Label reading is very important when purchasing prepared frozen meals, vegetables, and fruits. Most "complete" frozen dinners list sugar as an ingredient. One exception to this is the meals of the Weight Watchers brand, most of whose products appear to be sugar-free. Once again, it is far safer to quickly check the list of ingredients before purchasing any item.

Dressings, Relishes, and Sauces

Salad dressings, even the popular "low-cal" varieties all include sugar in their preparation. "Low-cal" simply means that a lower-than-normal quantity of sugar has been added. This decrease in refined sugar is usually compensated for by a sugar substitute such as sodium saccharin. Diet brands of salad dressings, such as Diamel and Tasti Diet, do not contain sugar at all, but instead use an artificial sweetener for flavoring. Tasti Diet's Italian dressing contains neither sugar nor its substitutes.

The list below indicates which of the most commonly used garnishes usually contain sugar and which usually do not.

Garnishes

Sugar-Free	*With Sugar*
dill pickles	barbecue sauce
horseradish	hamburger relish
horseradish mustard	ketchup
olives	mayonnaise
spicy brown mustard	salad dressings
Tabasco sauce	seafood cocktail sauce
yellow mustard	sweet pickles
	sweet relish
	tartar sauce
	Worcestershire sauce

Peanut Butter

The nutritional importance of peanut butter forces me to include it in a separate section. Peanuts are a very good source of protein and natural carbohydrates and so too is peanut butter. Ideally, it could be an outstanding snack, but unfortunately most easily accessible supermarket brands contain sugar. Just recently, however, I did find one brand of peanut butter in a large American supermarket that was completely natural and did not contain added sugar. You will find that the many health-food stores and nutritional centers always carry the more natural type of peanut butter. As most natural peanut butter is not homogenized, its oil tends to rise to the top of the jar—a situation easily remedied by simply stirring the peanut butter before using it. Some brands of natural peanut butter do not separate if kept in the refrigerator. I personally feel that the natural types of peanut butter have a better taste, more like fresh peanuts. These are becoming more plentiful and easier to obtain because of the recent increase in the number of nutritional centers, and the public's demand for more natural products.

Diet Foods

There is a special group of foods, found in most supermarkets and grocery stores, designed specifically for those who must limit their intake of sugar. Individuals who might purchase such products are diabetics and hypoglycemics who do not wish to drastically alter their well-established eating habits because of a metabolic disorder. Dieters might also purchase such products. These diet products include preserves, canned fruits and vegetables, salad dressings, gelatin desserts, and even ice cream. Many of them contain artificial sweeteners added to simulate the taste of their nondietetic equivalents. All of the preserves that I checked under dietetic labels did contain sugar substitutes. Details regarding the use of sugar substitutes by the migraine sufferer have already been explained in Chapter 10.

There are, in addition, some very good diet products that contain neither sugar nor its artificial substitutes. I found only one salad dressing in this category, an Italian dressing by Tasti Diet. Canned apricots, pears, fruit cocktail, peaches, and grapefruit sections can be found prepared in the juice provided them by nature (the same fruits are also available in syrup that is artificially sweetened). Most of the canned diet vegetables can be found without either sugar or its artificial substitutes.

Baby Foods

Baby-food companies in the early 1970s found themselves suffering from lowered sales, due in part to a trend toward homemade baby foods. The companies' remedy for this threat was to offer the cautious mothers an alternative. Many strained fruits and vegetables can now be found without any additives, sugar, or salt. For a family carrying a tendency to diabetes, hypoglycemia, or hypoglycemia complicated by migraine, this is an important breakthrough. If a child's pancreas is not abused from an early age by the constant stimulus of sugar-rich meals, there is a very good chance that he can avoid the discomforts of these sugar-related diseases later in life.

14

Conclusion

The purpose of this book is to inform the millions of persons suffering from the baffling problem of migraine that there is finally an answer for them. The answer is simple; it explains what is happening to them and how they can help themselves.

In the past, migraine victims have tried remedy after remedy, including the use of certain drugs that can themselves pose a very serious threat to health, since they may have dangerous side effects. The hazards connected with these drugs cannot be overemphasized, and the patient who takes them runs the risk of trading one form of ill health for another more serious ailment. The doctors who prescribe such drugs fully realize the problems involved in this type of therapy; however, until now, they had no other recourse in very serious cases of migraine.

Since stubborn cases of migraine have been mistakenly attributed to mental disorders, a great many headache sufferers have been sent to psychiatrists and psychoanalysts in search of a cure. The outcome of this course of therapy is invariably disheartening. Even after exhaustive sessions, which put a strain on both patience and pocketbook, the individual continues to be plagued by migraine, and becomes even more frustrated and despondent than before. Just how has the migraine victim become entangled in this seemingly endless and useless course of treatment? He is in this situation simply because of a fundamental mistake in connection with migraine. This mistake is the failure to understand that the patient's emotional disorders are not the cause of his headaches, and, furthermore, that his headaches are not the primary cause of his mental distress. The underlying, the basic, the true cause of all of his problems is the malfunctioning of his pancreas. Thus the only way permanently and effectively to break the vicious circle of migraine–emotional disease–migraine is to recognize the cause and eat properly. Any other approach to the problem is simply a concentrated effort to give temporary relief.

To control hyperinsulinism and prevent the blood sugar level from falling below normal, one need only apply the simple dietary therapy presented in the chapters of this book. The rules for this procedure are clear and easy to understand and need not be explained further. Two of them, however, deserve repeating. They are rules Number One and Number Two—completely eliminate refined sugar from the diet and never allow more than two to three hours to go by without eating. This therapy is the only sure way for a victim of migraine to rid himself of his headaches completely and permanently.

Since the ailment is chronic and relief requires continuous self-discipline, it is obvious that not just a remedy but a new way of life must be considered if the victim is to restore his health. The patient has a difficult decision to make. If he decides in favor of his health, he will be continually challenged to live up to this choice, because in order to accomplish his goal he must faithfully and daily adhere to his dietary regulations. He cannot go into this therapy halfheartedly, following the diet only when it is convenient, breaking his resolve when it is not, declaring that too many foods contain sugar in one form or another, or that it is too difficult to eat something every three hours. To fortify the commitment once it is made, the migraine patient can keep in mind certain important ideas: First is the sense of adventure and determination to win that this new undertaking will awaken. Another is the self-respect he will achieve if he manages to reach his goal. Still another is the knowledge that good habits can be formed as easily as bad ones, and that every exercise of willpower is another step toward establishing the way of life that will ultimately lead to complete relief from headaches. The success obtained by patients who have followed the recommendations set forth in the present work represents an overwhelming victory not only for the therapy recommended, but also for human intelligence, self-respect, and willpower. These patients prove that it is perfectly feasible to follow the advice given in this book, and that the success of the treatment is very real.

For the last twenty years, undoubtedly the best years of my life, I have daily adhered to the rules explained in this book. At first it was hard for me to give up my favorite sweets and sugared beverages, but little by little the feeling of deprivation faded as a new habit was being formed, bringing with it a sense of achievement and well-being. Today the new way of life is no longer new; it is settled habit. I no longer miss my old ways.

I am not the only one to have had such an experience. Others who have come to understand the nature of migraine and accepted my counseling have also proved capable of eliminating sugar from their diets. I want everyone to understand that the migraine patient need not continue to be a victim of this terrible ailment. With the help of his intelligence, imagination, and perseverance, he can rid himself of it and begin a normal, happier, and more rational life.

The way of life suggested in this book is a rational one because the individual accepts the situation and learns to control his role in it. The migraine sufferer will be able to increase his usefulness to society and to enjoy life more fully. It should not be forgotten, however, that it is also the duty of society to create conditions that will aid the individual in achieving his highest level of usefulness. I dare to hope that this book will challenge physicians and migraine sufferers to examine the evidence and confirm for themselves what I have described. I also dare to hope that by insisting on a more natural diet, and moving away from refined sugar, we may improve the quality of life in general—and bring the age-old migraine headache to extinction.

GLOSSARY

In order to facilitate comprehension of the text, definitions of some technical terms used in this book follow.

Acromegaly   Abnormality of growth characterized by excessive development of certain portions of the skeleton, particularly notable in the face and in the extremities.

Adrenaline   A hormone produced by the medulla of the adrenal glands, which plays an important role in carbohydrate metabolism. Adrenaline also dilates the air ducts, aiding respiration, and constricts the peripheral blood vessels, increasing blood pressure. It is also called epinephrine.

Allergy   Abnormal reaction of an organism in response to a foreign substance.

Arteriole   One of the small terminal branches of an artery that ends in capillaries.

Beriberi   A disease caused by a deficiency of thiamine, or vitamin B_1, characterized by weakness, wasting, and degenerative and inflammatory changes of the digestive system, the heart, and especially the nerves.

Biochemical Characterized by, produced by, or involving chemical reactions in living organisms.

Caffeine A bitter compound, found in coffee, tea, and kola nuts and used medicinally as a stimulant and diuretic. Caffeine stimulates the adrenal glands to produce adrenaline and other catecholamines.

Carbohydrate Essential substance in the nutrition of living beings, composed of carbon, hydrogen, and oxygen. Sugar and starch are carbohydrates.

Catecholamines Group of hormones secreted by the medulla of the adrenal glands; principal ones are adrenaline and noradrenaline.

Dextrose Another name for glucose.

Diabetes mellitus Disease caused by an insufficient production or utilization of insulin. It is characterized by an abnormally high concentration of glucose in the blood and by the presence of glucose in the urine, together with clinical symptoms.

Disaccharide A carbohydrate consisting of two molecules of simple sugars, or monosaccharides, chemically bound together.

Endocrine Pertaining to glands that produce hormones, also known as internal secretion glands.

Enzyme Organic substance that acts as a catalyst in the metabolic processes.

Epinephrine *See* Adrenaline.

Freeze-drying Drying process in which the water contained in a product is first frozen and then vaporized without passing through the liquid state, by the use of very low pressure.

Freeze-dried products completely recover their original properties when water is added to them. This process is also known as lyophilization.

Fructose A simple sugar, or monosaccharide, found in fruits, vegetables, and honey. It is the sweetest of all sugars. Fructose is also known as levulose, or fruit sugar.

Glucagon A hormone produced by the alpha cells of the islets of Langerhans in the pancreas. The action of glucagon is opposite to that of insulin: it increases the concentration of glucose in the blood by aiding the breakdown of glycogen.

Glucose The most important of all simple sugars, or monosaccharides, found in fruits, vegetables, and honey, and in small quantities in the blood of higher animals. Glucose is also known as dextrose and as grape sugar.

Glucose tolerance test A procedure to determine the amount of glucose in the blood.

Glycemia Quantity of glucose in the blood expressed in milligrams per 100 milliliters.

Glycogen Carbohydrate stored in the liver and in the muscles of the animal organism.

Glycogenic Referring to the formation of glycogen from glucose (glycogenesis) and to the breakdown of glycogen into glucose (glycogenolysis).

Gram Physical unit equal to the mass of one milliliter of distilled water at a temperature of 4° Centigrade. A gram is equivalent to about 1/28 ounce.

Hemianopsia Visual phenomenon characteristic of persons suffering from migraine; it consists in seeing only half of an object.

Hemicrania Unilateral headache.

Hormone Substance produced by the endocrine glands that regulates, stimulates, or inhibits the ability of the other organs to function properly.

Hydrolysis   Decomposition of a substance by the action of water.

Hyperglycemia   Above-normal concentration of glucose in the blood.

Hypoglycemia   Lower-than-normal concentration of glucose in the blood.

Hypoglycemic   A person who suffers from hypoglycemia; a drug or food that produces hypoglycemia.

Infantilism   Retention of childish physical, mental, or emotional qualities in adult life; especially, failure to attain sexual maturity.

Insulin   Hormone produced by the pancreas whose principal function is to metabolize glucose.

Internist   Medical doctor who is a specialist in internal medicine.

Intravenous   An intravenous injection is one that is made by puncturing a vein.

Islets of Langerhans   Patches of tissue in the pancreas consisting of special cells, the most important of which are the alpha and beta cells. The alpha cells produce the hormone glucagon and beta cells produce the hormone insulin. The islets of Langerhans also contain C cells and delta cells, the functions of which are unknown.

Lyophilization   *See* Freeze-drying.

Maltose   A disaccharide built of two molecules of glucose chemically linked together. It is found in corn syrup and in beer.

Metabolism   Chemical transformation that foods undergo in the organism in order to be utilized by it; also, other transformations that the constituent substances of the organism undergo to be converted into waste.

Microbe   An organism that is microscopic in size. This term is generally used to refer to a disease-causing microorganism.

Milligram One thousandth of a gram.

Molasses Dark brown syrup, containing 55 to 80 percent of sugar left over after crystallization of raw sugar.

Monosaccharide A carbohydrate that cannot be broken down into simpler substances that still retain the characteristic properties of carbohydrates, also called simple sugars. Glucose and fructose are examples of monosaccharides.

Night blindness A disease caused by deficiency of vitamin A; characterized by failure to see in the dark.

Noradrenaline A hormone produced by the medulla of the adrenal glands. Its effects are similar to those of adrenaline but less marked. Noradrenaline is also known as norepinephrine.

Norepinephrine *See* Noradrenaline.

Ophthalmic Pertaining to the eye.

Ophthalmologist A medical doctor, often a trained surgeon, who treats the troubles and diseases of the eyes.

Oxalic acid An organic acid found in small amounts in beer. It is a colorless, crystalline, and toxic compound.

Pancreas A compound gland that functions as an exocrine gland discharging digestive enzymes into the intestine and as an endocrine gland secreting insulin and glucagon into the bloodstream.

Pituitary A gland located in the base of the brain that internally secretes the growth hormone and several others whose primary functions are to stimulate the activity of the other glands. Also called the "master gland."

Prostaglandins A group of compounds produced by the body, similar to each other in chemical composition, that perform a great variety of functions in physiological processes. They have an effect on the caliber of the blood vessels and bronchi, act on the womb to produce childbirth and abortion, mediate in the immune response of the organism, etc. They also play an important role in the initiation of migraine attacks.

Royal jelly   Substance in honey that is fed by bees to the larvae. It is composed of carbohydrates, proteins, vitamins, and other not yet disclosed constituents.

Saccharin   A synthetic sweetener that has no nutritional value.

Scotomas   Scintillating luminous spots seen by some persons who suffer from migraine.

Scurvy   A disease caused by a deficiency of vitamin C, a nutrient found in many fruits, especially in citrus fruits. It is characterized by swollen gums, pain of the joints, anemia, and difficulty of wound healing. Scurvy is one of the oldest known diseases.

Starch   A carbohydrate that has a large molecule composed of many molecules of glucose chemically linked together. It is found in great quantities in cereals and potatoes, from which it is extracted commercially. Starch is the storage form of carbohydrates in plants.

Sucrose   A disaccharide composed of equal parts of glucose and fructose chemically bound together. It is found in many fruits and plants, especially in sugarcane and sugar beets, from which it is commercially extracted in great quantities.

Sugar beet   Sugar beet is second to sugarcane as a worldwide source of sugar. The sugar is stored in the root of the plant.

Sugarcane   A large perennial grass, belonging to the genus *Saccharum*, which grows only in a tropical humid climate. It is the principal source of the world's sugar production.

Thyroid   A gland located in the front part of the neck. It produces hormones that regulate metabolism, determine mental and physical development, and play a role in the functioning of the sex glands.

Tranquilizer A drug used to reduce anxiety and tension without impairing mental alertness.

Vasoconstrictor A substance that causes the blood vessels to constrict.

Vasodilator A substance that causes the blood vessels to dilate.

Venipuncture The insertion of a needle into a vein in order to withdraw blood or to administer intravenous feedings or medication.

Bibliography

Abrahamson, E. M., and Pezet, A. W. *Body, mind and sugar.* New York: Pyramid, 1971.

Allison, T. M. Migraine and acetonuria. *British Medical Journal* 1 (1927):165–66.

Amano, T., and Meyer, J. S. Prostaglandin inhibition and cerebrovascular control in patients with headache. *Headache* 22 (1982):52–59.

Anderson, J. W., and Herman, R. H. Treatment of reactive hypoglycemia with sulfonylureas. *American Journal of the Medical Sciences* 261 (1971):16–23.

Arcangeli, P. Headache, electric activity of the brain and blood sugar level: Clinical investigations of some correlative aspects of the problem. *Rivista di Neurobiologia* 4 (1958): 177–81.

Arcangeli, P., and Furian, R. Hypoglycemic headache. *Rivista Critica di Clinica Medica* 56 (1956):53–68.

Aretaeus. *The extant works of Aretaeus, the Cappadocian.* Edited and translated by Francis Adams. London: Printed for the Sydenham Society by Wertheimer and Co., 1856.

Arky, R. A. Pathophysiology and therapy of the fasting hypoglycemias. *Disease a Month* (Feb. 1968):1–47.

Asche, B. I., Mosenthal, H. O., and Ginsberg, G. Hypoglycemia with and without insulin, with and without symptoms. *Journal of Laboratory and Clinical Medicine* 13 (1927): 109–16.

Aykroyd, W. R. *The sweet malefactor: Sugar, slavery and human society*. London: Heinemann, 1967.

Bailey, H. *Vitamin E: Your key to a healthy heart*. New York: Arco, 1964.

Barnes, A. C. *The sugar cane—botany, cultivation and utilization*. London: Leonard Hill, 1964.

Barnett, H. L., Powers, J. R., Benward, J. H., et al. Salicylate intoxication in infants and children. *Journal of Pediatrics* 21 (1942):214–23.

Bergen, S. S., Jr., and Van Itallie, T. B. The glucagon problem. *New York Journal of Medicine* 61 (1961):779–86.

Bergström, S. Prostaglandins: Members of a new hormonal system. *Science* 157 (1967):382–91.

Bergström, S., and Sjövall, J. The isolation of prostaglandin E from sheep prostate glands. *Acta Chemica Scandinavica* 14 (1960):1701–5.

Black, J. Diazoxide and the treatment of hypoglycemia; an historical review. *Annals of the New York Academy of Sciences* 150 (1968):194–203.

Blau, J. N., and Cumings, J. N. Method of precipitating and preventing some migraine attacks. *British Medical Journal* 2 (1966):1242–43.

Blau, J. N., and Pyke, D. A. Effect of diabetes on migraine. *Lancet* 2 (1970):241–43.

Boonyaviroj, P., and Gutman, Y. Alpha-adrenergic stimulants, prostaglandins and catecholamine release from the adrenal gland in vitro. *Prostaglandins* 10 (1975):109–16.

———. Inhibition by PGE₂ and by phenylephrine of catecholamine release from human adrenal in vitro. *European Journal of Pharmacology* 41 (1977):73–75.

Brauch, F. Hypoglycemic headache. *Deutsche Medizinische Wohenschrift* 76 (1951):828–30.

Brunn, F. Contribution to the treatment of migraine. *Medizinische Klinik* 33 (1937):120–22.

Brunschwig, A., and Allen, J. G. Specific injurious action of alloxan upon pancreatic islet cells and convoluted tubules of the kidney: Comparative study in the rabbit, dog, and man. *Cancer Research* 4 (1944):45–54.

Buck, A. H. *The growth of medicine from the earliest times to about 1800.* New Haven: Yale University Press, 1917.

Cammidge, P. J. Chronic hypoglycaemia. *British Medical Journal* 1 (1930):818–22.

———. Chronic hypoglycaemia. *Practitioner* 119 (1927):102–12.

———. Hypoglycaemia. *Lancet* 2 (1924):1277–79.

———. Migraine and acetonuria. *British Medical Journal* 1 (1927):38–39.

Carlson, L. A., Ekelund, L. G., and Orö, L. Clinical and metabolic effects of different doses of prostaglandin E₁ in man: Prostaglandin and related factors. *Acta Medica Scandinavica* 183 (1968):423–30.

Chapleau, C. W., White, R. P., and Robertson, J. T. Cerebral vasodilation and prostacyclin. The effects of aspirin and meclofenamate in vitro. *Journal of Neurosurgery* 53 (1980):188–92.

Ciaccio, C., and Racchiusa, S. Effects of various sugars taken by mouth. *Bulletino della Societa Italiana di Biologia Sperimentale* 1 (1926):735–38.

Cleave, T. L., Campbell, G. D., Painter, N. S., et al. *Diabetes, coronary thrombosis, and the saccharine disease.* 2d ed. Bristol: John Wright & Sons, 1969.

Conn, J. W. The advantage of a high protein diet in the treatment of spontaneous hypoglycaemia. *Journal of Clinical Investigation* 15 (1936):673–78.

———. The diagnosis and management of spontaneous hypoglycemia. *Journal of the American Medical Association* 134 (1947):130–38.

Conn, J. W., and Seltzer, H. S. Spontaneous hypoglycemia. *American Journal of Medicine* 19 (1955):460–78.

Cotton, E. K., and Fahlberg, V. I. Hypoglycemia with salicylate poisoning. A report of two cases. *American Journal of the Diseases of Children* 108 (1964):171–73.

Critchley, M. The mechanism and treatment of migraine. *Practitioner* 133 (1934):54–61.

———. Prognosis in migraine. *Lancet* 2 (1936):35–36.

———. The treatment of migraine. *British Medical Journal* 2 (1935):794–96.

Critchley, M., and Ferguson, F. R. Migraine. Parts 1 and 2. *Lancet* 1 (1933):123–26, 183–87.

Deerr, N. *The history of sugar.* London: Chapman & Hall, 1949–1950.

Diamond, S., and Shapiro, D. B. "Long-term study of propranolol in the treatment of migraine." In *Advances in migraine research and therapy,* edited by F. C. Rose, 217–32. New York: Raven Press, 1982.

Dollery, C. T., Pentecost, B. L., Samaan, N. A., et al. Drug-induced diabetes. *Lancet* 2 (1962):735–37.

Dublin, L. I. *Factbook on man: From birth to death.* 2d ed. New York: Macmillan, 1965.

Dufty, W. *Sugar blues.* New York: Warner Books, 1976.

Dunn, R. S. *Sugar and slaves: The rise of the planter class in the English West Indies, 1624–1713.* Chapel Hill: University of North Carolina Press, 1972.

Ellis, E. D. *An introduction to the history of sugar as a commodity.* Philadelphia: J. C. Winston, 1905.

Elrick, H., Staub, A., and Maske, H. Recent developments in glucagon research. *New England Journal of Medicine* 256 (1957):742–47.

Fabrykant, M., and Bruger, M. Dynamics of the hypoglycemic reaction. *American Journal of the Medical Sciences* 216 (1948):84–95.

Fajans, S. S., Floyd, J. C., Jr., Thiffault, C. A., et al. Further studies on diazoxide suppression of insulin release from abnormal islet tissue in man. *Annals of the New York Academy of Sciences* 150 (1968):261–80.

Fawkes, M. Migraine and acetonuria. *British Medical Journal* 2 (1926):1176–78.

Feuerstein, N., Feuerstein, G., and Gutman, Y. Endogenous prostaglandins modulate adrenal catecholamine secretion. *European Journal of Pharmacology* 58 (1979):489–92.

Field, J. B., Boyle, C., Remer, A., et al. Clinical and physiologic studies using diazoxide in the treatment of hypoglycemia. *Annals of the New York Academy of Sciences* 150 (1968):415–28.

Flower, R., Gryglewski, R., Herbaczynska-Cedro, K., et al. Effects of anti-inflammatory drugs on prostaglandin biosynthesis. *Nature (New Biology)* 238 (1972):104–6.

Flower, R., and Vane, J. R. Inhibition of prostaglandin synthetase in brain explains the anti-pyretic activity of paracetamol (4-acetamidophenol). *Nature* (London) 240 (1972):410–11.

Foldes, E. Migraine therapy by diet poor in carbohydrates. *Klinische Wochenschrift* 18 (1939):390–91.

Fredericks, C., and Goodman, H. *Low blood sugar and you*. New York: Constellation International, 1969.

Freinkel, N., Arky, R. A., Singer, D. L., et al. Alcohol hypoglycemia. Part 4: Current concepts of its pathogenesis. *Diabetes* 14 (1965):350–61.

Friede, K. H. Symptomatology and differential diagnosis of hypoglycemia. *Medizinische Klinik* 50 (1955):1739–40.

Friedman, A. P. Symposium on headaches and related pain syndromes. *Medical Clinics of North America* 62 (1978):427–623.

Friedman, A. P., et al. Observations on vascular headache of the migraine type. In *Background to migraine*, edited by J. N. Cumings. London: Whitefriars Press, 1973.

Gabrielian, E. S., and Amroian, E. A. Response of cerebral vessels to noradrenaline under hypocapnic condition and inhibition of prostaglandin biosynthesis. *Biulleten Eksperimentalnoi Biologii i Meditsiny* 81 (1976):643–45.

Geerlings, H. C. P. *The world's cane sugar industry, past and present*. Manchester: N. R. Altrincham, 1912.

Gilgore, S. G. The influence of salicylate on hyperglycemia. *Diabetes* 9 (1960):392–93.

Gillam, D. M., and Harper, J. R. Hypoglycaemia after alcohol ingestion. *Lancet* 1 (1973):829–30.

Girard, J., and Colleson, L. Migraine and glycemic perturbations. *Presse Medicale* 37 (1939):705–8.

Graber, A. L., Porte, D., Jr., and Williams, R. H. Clinical use of diazoxide and mechanisms for its hyperglycemic effects. *Diabetes* 15 (1966):143–48.

———. Mechanisms of diazoxide hyperglycemia. *Diabetes* 14 (1965):450–54.

Gray, P. A., and Burtness, H. L. Hypoglycemic headache. *Endocrinology* 19 (1935):549–60.

Griffith, J. E., Jr., Jackson, R. L., and Janes, R. G. Action of alloxan on a hypoglycemic infant. *Pediatrics* 7 (1951): 616–22.

Hamberg, M., and Samuelsson, B. On the metabolism of prostaglandins E₁ and E₂ in man. *Journal of Biological Chemistry* 246 (1971):6713–21.

Hamberg, M., Svensson, J., and Samuelsson, B. Thromboxanes: A new group of biologically active compounds derived from prostaglandin endoperoxides. *Proceedings of the National Academy of Sciences of the United States* 72 (1975):2994–98.

Harell, A., Laurian, L., Ayalon, D., et al. Hypoglycemia due to hyperinsulinism treated by streptozotocin and diazoxide. *Israel Journal of Medical Sciences* 8 (1972):895–96.

Harnapp, G. O. Hyperinsulinism. *Monatsschrift der Kinderheilkunde* 65 (1936):407–25.

Harrill, J. A. Headache and vertigo associated with hypoglycemic tendency. *Laryngoscope* 61 (1951):138–45.

Harris, S. The diagnosis and treatment of hyperinsulinism. *Annals of Internal Medicine* 10 (1936):514–33.

———. Hyperinsulinism. *Southern Medical Journal* 37 (1944):714–17.

———. Hyperinsulinism, a definite disease entity: Etiology, pathology, symptoms, diagnosis, prognosis and treatment of spontaneous insulogenic hypoglycemia (hyperinsulinism). *Journal of the American Medical Association* 101 (1933):1958–65.

———. Hyperinsulinism and dysinsulinism. *Journal of the American Medical Association* 83 (1924):729–33.

Hartmann, F. L. Hypoglycemia. *Medical Clinics of North America* 12 (1929):1035–39.

Hay, K. M. *Do something about that migraine.* London: Tandem Books, 1968.

Hecht, A., and Goldner, M. G. Reappraisal of the hypoglycemic action of acetylsalicylate. *Metabolism: Clinical and Experimental* 8 (1959):418–28.

Hinman, J. W. Prostaglandins. *Annual Review of Biochemistry* 41 (1972):161–78.

Horne, W. D. Sugar industries of the United States. *Industrial and Engineering Chemistry* 27 (1935):989–95.

Hunt, T. C. Bilious migraine. *Lancet* 2 (1933):279–85.

Jordan, S. M. Relationship of migraine to functional colon disease. *Transactions of the American Gastroenterological Association* 31 (1929):332–36.

Jordan, W. R. Neurological manifestations of hypoglycemia. *New England Journal of Medicine* 209 (1933):715–19.

Katsh, G. On the prediabetic phase of diabetes. *Deutsche Medizinische Wochenschrift* 75 (1950):1331–32.

———. The processes of metabolism. *Munchener Medizinische Wochenschrift* 101 (1959):65–70.

Knaggs, H. V. *The truth about sugar.* London: C. W. Daniel, 1913.

Korbut, R. Bioassay of prostaglandins in the presence of high concentrations of catecholamines. *Polish Journal of Pharmacology and Pharmacy* 27 (1975):631–36.

Kvam, D. C., and Stanton, H. C. Studies on diazoxide hyperglycemia. *Diabetes* 13 (1964):639–44.

Lake, G. B. Hyperinsulinism. *Clinical Medicine and Surgery* 42 (1935):316–17.

Laroche, G. The spontaneous hypoglycemias. *Semaine des Hopitaux de Paris* 23 (1947):2165–73.

Limbeck, G. A., Ruvalcaba, R. H. A., Samols, E., et al. Salicylates and hypoglycemia. *American Journal of the Diseases of Children* 109 (1965):165–67.

Ljungström, B. Glucagon treatment in spontaneous hypoglycemia. *Nordisk Medicin* 71 (1964):177–79.

Low, R. Migraine and hypoglycemia. *Tribuna Medica* (Colombia) 655 (1977):35–40.

Low, R., and Casas, M. C. The flat glucose tolerance curve. *Tribuna Medica* (Colombia) 653 (1977):25–26.

———. Insulin response to different refined and unrefined carbohydrates. *Tribuna Medica* (Colombia) 652 (1977): 30–32.

———. Tolerance tests with different refined and unrefined carbohydrates. *Tribuna Medica* (Colombia) 651 (1977): 27–29.

Magill, C. D. Another treatment for migraine headache. *Journal of the American Medical Association* 222 (1972):703–4.

Major, R. H., ed. *Classic descriptions of disease with biographical sketches of the authors.* Springfield, Ill.: C. C. Thomas, 1932.

Malvea, B. P., Gwon, N., and Graham, J. R. Propranolol prophylaxis of migraine. *Headache* 12 (1973):163–67.

Marks, V., and Samols, E. Diazoxide therapy of intractable hypoglycemia. *Annals of the New York Academy of Sciences* 150 (1968):442–54.

Martindale, W. *The extra pharmacopoeia.* 26th ed. London: Pharmaceutical Press, 1972.

Marx, H. Spontaneous hypoglycemia. *Deutsche Medizinische Wochenschrift* 62 (1936):843–47.

Mayhew, D., Wright, P. H., and Ashmore, J. Regulation of insulin secretion. *Pharmacological Review* 21 (1969):183–212.

Mereu, T. R., Kassoff, A., and Goodman, A. D. Diazoxide in

the treatment of infantile hypoglycemia. *New England Journal of Medicine* 275 (1966):1455–60.

Messina, E. J., Weiner, R., and Kaley, G. Inhibition of bradykinin vasodilation and potentiation of norepinephrine and angiotensin vasoconstriction by inhibitors of prostaglandin synthesis in skeletal muscle of the rat. *Circulation Research* 37 (1975):430–37.

Metz, S. A., Fujimoto, W. Y., and Robertson, R. P. Modulation of insulin secretion by cyclic AMP and prostaglandin E: the effects of theophylline, sodium salicylate and tolbutamide. *Metabolism* 31 (1982):1014–22.

————. A role for prostaglandins as mediators of alpha-adrenergic inhibition of the acute insulin response to glucose. *Advances in Prostaglandin Thromboxane and Leukotrien Research* 8 (1980):1291–94.

Meythaler, F., and Ehrmann-Rostock, M. Spontaneous hypoglycemia. *Ergebnisse der Inneren Medizin und Kinderheilkunde* 54 (1938):116–43.

Miller, J. B. Hypoglycaemic effect of oxytetracycline. *British Medical Journal* 2 (1966):1007–9.

Minot, G. R. The role of a low carbohydrate diet in the treatment of migraine and headache. *Medical Clinics of North America* 7 (1923):715–28.

Mitchell, M. L., Ernesti, M., Raben, M. S., et al. Control of hypoglycemia with diazoxide and hormones. *Annals of the New York Academy of Sciences* 150 (1968):406–14.

Moench, L. G. *Headache*. Chicago: Yearbook Publishers, 1947.

Molinier, A., Maugard, A., and Tchourumoff, N. Study of blood sugar changes in alcoholics. *Semaine des Hopitaux de Paris* 42 (1966):1569–78.

Moretti, R. L., and Abraham, S. Stimulation of microsomal prostaglandin synthesis by a vasoactive material isolated from blood plasma. *Prostaglandins* 15 (1978):603–22.

Morgan, C. R., and Lazarow, A. Immunoassay of insulin: Two

antibody system. Plasma insulin levels of normal, subdiabetic and diabetic rats. *Diabetes* 12 (1963):115–26.

Nasjletti, A., and Malik, K. U. Interrelations between prostaglandins and vasoconstrictor hormones: Contributions to blood pressure regulation. *Federation Proceedings* 41 (1982):2394–99.

Nelson, N. A photometric adaptation of the Somogyi method for the determination of glucose. *Journal of Biological Chemistry* 153 (1944):375–80.

Newman, W. P., and Brodows, R. G. Metabolic effects of prostaglandin E_2 infusion in man: Possible adrenergic mediation. *Journal of Clinical Endocrinology and Metabolism* 55 (1982):496–501.

Pearce, J. Insulin induced hypoglycaemia in migraine. *Journal of Neurology, Neurosurgery and Psychiatry* 34 (1971):154–56.
———. *Migraine: Clinical features, mechanisms and management.* Springfield, Ill.: C. C. Thomas, 1969.

Pennink, M., White, R. P., Crockarell, J. R., et al. Role of prostaglandin F_2 in the genesis of experimental cerebral vasospasm. *Journal of Neurosurgery* 37 (1972):398–406.

Pickles, V. R., Hall, W. J., Best, F. A., et al. Prostaglandins in endometrium and menstrual fluid from normal and dysmenorrhoeic subjects. *British Journal of Obstetrics and Gynaecology* 72 (1965):185–92.

Pike, J. R. Prostaglandins. *Scientific American* 225 (1971): 84–92.

Porges, O. Treatment of migraine by carbohydrate restriction. *Medizinische Klinik* 33 (1937):664–65.

Porte, D., Jr. Inhibition of insulin release by diazoxide and its relation to catecholamine effects in man. *Annals of the New York Academy of Sciences* 150 (1968):281–91.

Portis, S. A. Life situations, emotions and hyperinsulinism. *Journal of the American Medical Association* 142 (1950):1281–86.

Powell, E. Cerebral malnutrition and mental malfunction. *Medical Record* 144 (1936):318–22.

————. Does normal mental function depend on normal blood sugar? *Tri-State Medical Journal* 7 (1935):1421–28.

————. The role of diet in the etiology and treatment of mental disease resulting from hyperinsulinism. *Tri-State Medical Journal* 6 (1934):1323–27.

Ramwell, P. W. *The prostaglandins.* 3 vols. New York: Plenum Press, 1978–1980.

Reed, W. *The history of sugar and sugar yielding plants together with an epitome of every notable process of sugar extraction.* London: Longmans Green, 1866.

Reid, J., and Lightbody, T. D. The insulin equivalence of salicylate. *British Medical Journal* 1 (1959):897–900.

Roberts, H. J. Migraine and related vascular headaches due to diabetogenic hyperinsulinism: Observations on pathogenesis and rational treatment in 421 patients. *Headache* 7 (1967):41–62.

Robertson, R. P., Gavarenski, D. J., Porte, D., et al. Inhibition of in vivo insulin secretion by prostaglandin E_1. *Journal of Clinical Investigation* 54 (1974):310–15.

Robinson, H. J., and Vane, J. R., eds. *Prostaglandin synthesis inhibitors—their effects on physiological functions and pathological states.* New York: Raven Press, 1974.

Rosdahl, N. Hyperinsulinism treated with diazoxide. *Ugeskrift for Laeger* 131 (1969):1698–701.

Rosenblum, W. I. Effects of prostaglandins on cerebral blood vessels: Interaction with vasoactive amines. *Neurology* (Minneapolis) 25 (1975):1169–71.

Rubenstein, A. H., Levin, N. W., and Elliott, G. A. Manganese-induced hypoglycaemia. *Lancet* 2 (1962):1348–51.

Ruvalcaba, R. H. A., Limbeck, G. A., and Kelley, V. C. Acetaminophen and hypoglycemia. *American Journal of the Diseases of Children* 112 (1966):558–60.

Rynaersch, E. H., and Moersch, F. P. Neurologic manifestations of hyperinsulinism and other hypoglycemic states. *Journal of the American Medical Association* 103 (1934):1196–99.

Samuelsson, B., Goldyne, M., Granström, E., et al. Prostaglandins and thromboxanes. *Annual Review of Biochemistry* 47 (1978):997–1029.

Samuelsson, B., Granström, E., Green, K., et al. Prostaglandins. *Annual Review of Biochemistry* 44 (1975):669–95.

Samuelsson, B., Ramwell, P., and Paoletti, R. *Advances in prostaglandin and thromboxane research.* New York: Raven Press, 1980.

Schnitker, M. T., and Schnitker, M. A. A clinical test for migraine. *Journal of the American Medical Association* 135 (1947):89–91.

Seltzer, H. S. Drug-induced hypoglycemia: A review based on 473 cases. *Diabetes* 21 (1972):955–66.

Seltzer, H. S., and Allen, E. W. Hyperglycemia and inhibition of insulin secretion during administration of diazoxide and trichlormethiazide in man. *Diabetes* 18 (1969):19–28.

Seltzer, H. S., Allen, E. W., Herron, A. L., et al. Insulin secretion in response to glycemic stimulus: Relation of delayed initial response to carbohydrate intolerance in mild diabetes mellitus. *Journal of Clinical Investigation* 46 (1967):323–35.

Seltzer, H. S., and Crout, J. R. Insulin secretory blockade by benzothiadiazines and catecholamines; reversal by sulfonylureas. *Annals of the New York Academy of Sciences* 150 (1968):309–21.

Seltzer, H. S., Fajans, S. S., and Conn, J. W. Spontaneous hypoglycemia as an early manifestation of diabetes mellitus. *Diabetes* 5 (1956):437–42.

Simon, E., Frenkel, G., and Kraicer, P. F. Blockade of insulin secretion by mannoheptulose. *Israel Journal of Medical Sciences* 8 (1972):743–52.

Skinner, W., and Madison, L. L. A new role of glucagon and epinephrine in producing their counter-regulatory response to hypoglycemia. *Clinical Research* 8 (1960):247–52.

Smith, H. M. Diazoxide in the treatment of hypoglycemia. *Annals of the New York Academy of Sciences* 150 (1968): 191–97.

Sokol, J. E. Glucagon—an essential hormone. *American Journal of Medicine* 41 (1966):331–41.

Soskin, S. Role of the endocrines in the regulation of blood sugar. *Journal of Clinical Endocrinology* 4 (1944):75–88.

Southwell, N., Williams, J. D., and Mackenzie, I. Methysergide in the prophylaxis of migraine. *Lancet* 1 (1964): 523–24.

Spengler, F. Causes and manifestations of hypoglycemia. *Munchener Medizinische Wochenschrift* 84 (1937):2015–16.

Spira, P. J., Mylecharane, E. J., Misbach, J., et al. Internal and external carotid vascular responses to vasoactive agents in the monkey. *Neurology* (Minneapolis) 28 (1978):162–73.

Steigerwaldt, F. Glucagon in hypoglycemic conditions. *Medizinische Klinik* 61 (1966):1585–87.

Strong, L. A. G. *The story of sugar.* London: Weidenfeld and Nicolson, 1954.

Sussman, K. E., Stimmler, L., and Birenboim, H. Plasma insulin levels during reactive hypoglycemia. *Diabetes* 15 (1966):1–4.

Sutton, J. A. Diabetes and migraine. *Lancet* 2 (1970):570–71.

Talbot, N. B., Crawford, J. D., and Bailey, C. C. Use of mesoxalyl-urea (alloxan) in the treatment of infant with convulsions due to idiopathic hypoglycemia. *Pediatrics* 1 (1948):337–45.

Tidy, H. L. *A synopsis of medicine.* 8th ed. Bristol: John Wright & Sons, 1945.

Umber, F. Hypoglycemia in practice. *Deutsche Medizinische Wochenschrift* 68 (1942):261–67.

United Nations. *Statistical yearbook, 1981.* New York: United Nations, 1981.

United States Beet Sugar Association. *The beet sugar story.* 3d ed. Washington, D.C., 1959.

United States Bureau of Census. *Statistical abstract of the United States, 1984.* Washington, D.C., 1984.

Vachon, A., Noel, G., Gauthier, J., et al. Current drug therapy of organic hypoglycemia. *Lyon Medical* 220 (1968):399–409.

Vane, J. R. Inhibition of prostaglandin synthesis as a mechanism of action for aspirin-like drugs. *Nature (New Biology)* 231 (1971):232–35.

Vane, J. R., and Ferreira, S. H. "Anti-inflammatory drugs." In *Handbook of experimental pharmacology.* New York: Springer Verlag, 1979.

Vierhapper, H., Grubeck-Loebenstein, B., Korn, A., et al. Release and vasoactive actions of catecholamines during inhibition of prostaglandin synthesis in normal man. *Hypertension* 4 (1982):112–17.

Viinikka, L., and Ylikorkala, O. Effect of various doses of acetylsalicylic acid in combination with dipyridamole on the balance between prostacyclin and thromboxane in human serum. *British Journal of Pharmacology* 72 (1981):299–303.

Wagner-Jauregg, J. Degenerative migraine and its treatment. *Wiener Medizinische Wochenschrift* 85 (1935):1–9.

Waters, W. C. Spontaneous hypoglycemia: Role of diet in etiology and treatment. *Southern Medical Journal* 24 (1931): 249–52.

Watson, G. *Nutrition and your mind: The psychochemical response.* New York: Harper & Row, 1972.

Weber, R. B., and Reinmuth, O. M. The treatment of migraine with propranolol. *Neurology* 22 (1972):366–69.

Welch, K. M., Spira, P. J., Knowles, L., et al. Effects of prostaglandins on the internal and external carotid blood flow in the monkey: Possible relevance to cranial flow changes during migraine headache. *Neurology* (Minneapolis) 24 (1974):705–10.

Whitehouse, F. W. Glucagon for hypoglycemia. *Journal of the Michigan Medical Society* 61 (1962):1221.

Wideroe, T. E., and Vigander, T. Propranolol in the treatment of migraine. *British Medical Journal* 2 (1974):699–701.

Wilder, J. Problems of spontaneous hypoglycemia. *Zeitschrift fur die Gesamte Experimentelle Medizin* 76 (1931):136–57.

Wilder, R. M. Hyperinsulinism. *International Clinics* 2 (1933): 1–18.

———. Spontaneous hypoglycemia. *International Clinics* 3 (1936):143–63.

Wilkinson, C. F., Jr. Recurrent migrainoid headaches associated with spontaneous hypoglycemia. *American Journal of the Medical Sciences* 218 (1949):209–12.

Winton, A. L., and Winton, K. G. *The structure and composition of foods.* Vol 2. New York: J. Wiley & Sons, 1935.

Wolff, G. Hypoglycemia. *Medizinische Monatsschrift* 24 (1970):297–300.

Wolff, H. G. *Headache and other head pain.* 2d ed. New York: Oxford University Press, 1963.

Yalow, R. S., and Berson, S. A. Dynamics of insulin secretion in hypoglycemia. *Diabetes* 14 (1965):341–49.
————. Immunoassay of endogenous plasma insulin in man. *Journal of Clinical Investigation* 39 (1960):1157–75.

Zarafonetis, C. J. D. Therapeutic possibilities of para-amino-benzoic acid. *Annals of Internal Medicine* 30 (1949):1188–211.
Zivin, I. The neurological and psychiatric aspects of hypoglycemia. *Diseases of the Nervous System* 31 (1970):604–7.

Index

About the Author

Rodolfo Low was born in Barmen, Germany, in 1912, but spent most of his early life in Spain. It was there that he earned his undergraduate degree in chemistry in 1935. He then returned to Germany to work toward his Ph.D.

In 1937 he went to South America as a professor at the National University of Colombia, where he taught physical chemistry and other subjects. From 1949 until 1951 he held the position of dean of sciences.

In 1957 Professor Low was appointed president of the University of Santander in Bucaramanga, Colombia, a position that he held until 1962. He acted as Ford Foundation adviser in higher education until 1965 and as Ford Foundation adviser in science and technology until 1975.

He initiated his research on migraine in 1961, while he was still university president, and continued it during the years he was adviser for the Ford Foundation. Most of the experimental part of his research was carried out in the laboratory of biochemistry at the Pontifical Catholic University in Bogotá. The insulin determinations were done at the laboratory of nuclear medicine at the University of Antioquia in Medellín, Colombia. He applied the results of his research to hundreds of migraine sufferers with great success.

In 1983 he came to the United States and repeated his research and testing at the medical offices of Dr. Fredric W. Pullen II in Miami, Florida, with the same extraordinary results. The effectiveness of his treatment has also been validated by the Department of Neurology at Bowman Gray School of Medicine, Wake Forest University, Winston-Salem, North Carolina.